Flesh and Bones of
PATHOLOGY

To Mandy, Charlotte and Harry for their love and support, as always
ACB

To my parents, in appreciation of a lifetime of love and support
NJC

Commissioning Editor: **Timothy Horne**
Development Editor: **Barbara Simmons**
Copy Editor: **Jane Ward**
Project Manager: **Frances Affleck**
Designer: **Stewart Larking**
Illustration Manager: **Merlyn Harvey**

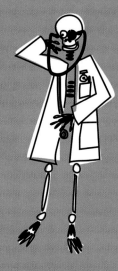

Flesh and Bones of
PATHOLOGY

Adrian Bateman BSc MD FRCPath
Consultant Histopathologist
Southampton University Hospitals NHS Trust;
Honorary Senior Lecturer in Pathology
University of Southampton, UK

Norman Carr MB BS FRCPath FRCPA
Professor of Anatomical Pathology
Graduate School of Medicine
University of Wollongong
New South Wales, Australia

Illustrations by Jennifer Rose

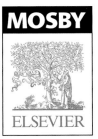

MOSBY

ELSEVIER

Edinburgh   London   New York   Oxford   Philadelphia   St Louis   Sydney   Toronto   2009

MOSBY
ELSEVIER

First published 2009

ISBN 978-0-7234-3396-5

British Library Cataloguing in Publication Data
A catalogue record for this book is available from the British Library

Library of Congress Cataloging in Publication Data
A catalog record for this book is available from the Library of Congress

Notice:
Neither the Publisher nor the Authors assume any responsibility for any loss or injury and/or damage to persons or property arising out of or related to any use of the material contained in this book. It is the responsibility of the treating practitioner, relying on independent expertise and knowledge of the patient, to determine the best treatment and method of application for the patient.
The Publisher

The
publisher's
policy is to use
**paper manufactured
from sustainable forests**

Working together to grow
libraries in developing countries

www.elsevier.com | www.bookaid.org | www.sabre.org

ELSEVIER   BOOK AID
            International   Sabre Foundation

ELSEVIER   your source for books,
            journals and multimedia
            in the health sciences
www.elsevierhealth.com

Printed in China

Contents

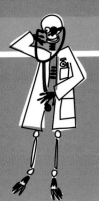

The big picture

Pathology is unusual in that it can be viewed as a core basic medical science and as a range of clinical specialties. Pathology as a basic academic subject is the study and understanding of disease processes. A thorough knowledge of pathology, therefore, underpins the study of clinical medicine. Pathology as a clinical specialty is the use of scientific methods to investigate the causes and effects of disease within the body—in particular, the structural and functional changes that occur in cells and tissues in response to injuries, abnormal stimuli or genetic abnormalities, and their consequences for the organism as a whole. Clinicians within almost every branch of medicine interact with clinical pathology services; consequently, it is very important that the student understands the role of pathology specialties in patient management, whether or not a career in pathology is being considered!

The aim of this book is to instil a broad working knowledge of pathology as relevant to current clinical medicine. The book is not intended as a fully comprehensive reference text—there are several other volumes that perform this function admirably—but as a 'checklist' of the most important concepts within pathology that facilitate intellectual links between disease processes at the cellular and clinical levels.

This section sets the scene by defining the term pathology and describing the roles of this subject both as a basic medical science and as a clinical speciality. It is followed by the 'High return facts'—a checklist of the most important pathology-based concepts. Each one of these is expanded into more detail in Section three, which uses a double-page format with simple figures wherever possible to facilitate the learning process.

■ WHAT IS PATHOLOGY?

The word 'pathology' is derived from the Greek *pathos*, suffering, and *logos*, study. It uses scientific methods to investigate the causes and effects of disease within the body, in particular the structural and functional changes that occur in cells and tissues in response to injuries, abnormal stimuli or genetic abnormalities, and their consequences for the organism as a whole.

As a clinical subject pathology grew up

■ in the postmortem dissecting room where autopsies revealed the morphological changes associated with disease (morbid anatomy); the word autopsy comes from the Greek word for eyewitness and can be translated as 'seeing for oneself'

■ in side-rooms adjacent to hospital wards, in which doctors, nurses and medical students could carry out simple diagnostic tests.

As the number and complexity of tests grew, a centralized laboratory was set up in each hospital with dedicated technical staff. The work of the hospital laboratory continued to expand until it required the attention of a full-time specialist: the pathologist.

In the UK, pathology is nowadays divided into a number of disciplines, each with its own specialist practitioners:

■ **cellular pathology** (**histopathology**): structural changes in diseased tissues are examined macroscopically or microscopically; this is the focus of the remainder of this book and the use of the term 'pathology' from this section on refers mainly to cellular pathology

■ **clinical chemistry** or **chemical pathology**: metabolic disturbances are investigated, mainly by changes in the concentration of substances in body fluids

■ **haematology**: diseases of the blood and bone marrow

■ **microbiology**: detection and characterization of bacteria, viruses, fungi and parasites

■ **immunology**: abnormalities of the immune system

■ **medical genetics**: the inheritance of disease.

Pathology has a central place in modern medical practice. On the one hand, it represents the conceptual framework by which healthcare professionals organize their understanding of disease processes. Advances in clinical and basic science research are constantly modifying this understanding. On the other hand, laboratory tests are a vital part of the diagnosis of a wide range of diseases. Thus, pathology represents the link between the patient and the laboratory.

■ LABORATORY TECHNIQUES WITHIN CELLULAR PATHOLOGY

Macroscopic and microscopic assessment of specimens

Most small biopsies obtained with a biopsy needle (e.g. needle biopsies from breast or prostate) or at endoscopy (e.g. gastric, colonic and bronchial biopsies) may be 'processed' in their entirety into paraffin wax tissue blocks (see below). However, larger specimens (e.g. from a small ellipse of skin to an entire organ) do not need to be processed in their totality in order to reach a diagnosis. With these larger specimens, accurate diagnosis relies on naked eye (macroscopic) examination of specimens, with recording of the most important anatomical and pathological features and careful choice of tissue *samples* for processing and microscopic assessment.

Tissue processing

The formalin-preserved tissue from which thin sections are to be made for microscopic examination is placed into small plastic containers termed 'processing cassettes'. Each cassette can contain tissue up to approximately $20\,mm \times 20\,mm$ in area and up to $4\,mm$ in thickness. Using an automated machine that usually works during the night, these tissue fragments are dehydrated and then impregnated with paraffin wax before being manually orientated correctly within a solid block of wax (embedding). This imparts stiffness to the tissues and enables very thin sections, typically 4–$5\,\mu m$, to be cut manually from the tissue blocks and placed on to glass microscope slides. These thin sections are then dewaxed prior to staining and a thin glass cover slip is placed over the section to protect the delicate tissue. The glass slides with attached sections are then ready for viewing under a light microscope. Glass microscope slides and tissue blocks effectively form part of patients' medical records and are kept for many years within archived hospital stores in case further examination is required.

Routine histochemical stains

Tissues require staining in order to allow visualization with a microscope—unstained tissue sections are almost invisible. The most common routine combination of tissue stains is haematoxylin and eosin (H&E). Haematoxylin is a basic dye that binds to structures including DNA and, therefore, stains nuclei blue. Eosin stains cytoplasm and extracellular structures such as collagen and basement membranes in shades of red. A diagnosis can be achieved in the majority of tissue sections after examination of the H&E stain alone. There is a large range of additional histochemical stains, each demonstrating different cellular and extracellular components through specific chemical reactions that are induced within the tissue sections. For example, mucin and glycogen are stained purple using the periodic acid–Schiff method.

Immunohistochemistry

While histochemical stains are very useful, immunohistochemistry is a more sensitive and specific method for demonstrating the presence of substances within a tissue section. Since its introduction to diagnostic cellular pathology in the 1980s, immunohistochemistry has become an essential tool within the modern laboratory. The technique relies on identification of a cellular or extracellular tissue component using immune binding of a specially prepared antibody solution to a corresponding antigen within a tissue section. The bound and immobilized antibody is visualized using a chemical reaction involving a dye, which reveals the presence of the antigen within the tissue section. Examples of the use of immunohistochemistry in diagnostic cellular pathology include the accurate typing of tumours, the assessment of the likely rate of cell division within a tissue and the identification of microorganisms such as bacteria and viruses.

Electron microscopy

Conventional light microscopy may be used to magnify images of stained tissue up to 1000 times, which is sufficient for most diagnostic requirements. However, tissues can be viewed under much greater magnifications (e.g. up to 10 000–25 000 times) using the electron microscope because electrons have a much shorter wavelength than visible light. In transmission electron microscopy, a 'shadow image' is created by firing electrons at a very thin plastic-embedded tissue section within a vacuum. This technique is most commonly used today within diagnostic cellular pathology for the examination of glomeruli within renal biopsies, although other uses include the diagnosis of unusual tumours.

Molecular techniques

Research is continually leading to a greater understanding of the alterations in nucleic acids that occur during the development and progression of disease. Two investigative techniques that are extremely useful for studying nucleic acids during the diagnostic process in cellular pathology are the **polymerase chain reaction (PCR)** and **in-situ hybridization**. PCR is a powerful method for increasing the quantity of DNA available for subsequent analysis and is usually performed using DNA extracted from blood or stored tissues. Modified PCR-based methods may be used, for example, to search for mutations as a means of identifying the development of tumours such as lymphoma or to confirm the diagnosis of certain unusual but important tumours based on characteristic genetic alterations. In-situ hybridization identifies specific nucleic acids *within* tissue sections using specific nucleic acid 'probes', which bind to (i.e. attach strongly to) a corresponding nucleic acid 'target', if present, within a section. Identification of bound probes within a tissue section is achieved either using a dye that is visible using conventional light microscopy or a dye that fluoresces when illuminated by ultraviolet light (fluorescence in-situ hybridization (FISH)). Examples of the use of in-situ hybridization within diagnostic cellular pathology would be the confirmation of certain types of viral infection (e.g. Epstein–Barr virus) using dyes visible with conventional microscopy or the identification of multiple copies of the gene HER-2 in breast cancer using a fluorescent probe.

Cytopathology

Cytopathology is the examination of preparations in which cells have become dissociated from each other. Whereas histological sections show the architecture of tissues and organs, cytological preparations do not. For example, cervical smears are cytological preparations. A spatula or brush is used to scrape cells from the uterine cervix; these are spread on a slide, and then the cells are examined under the light microscope to look for changes that may indicate the presence of neoplasia. Other examples of cytopathology are the examination of desquamated cells in fluids such as urine or effusions, and fine needle aspiration cytology in which cells are extracted from suspected tumours using a needle and syringe. Histochemical stains, immunohistochemical techniques and molecular biological methods may all be used with cytological material.

■ PATHOLOGY: A BASIC MEDICAL SCIENCE OR A CLINICAL SPECIALTY?

Pathology is unique within medicine as a subject that is considered a basic medical science as well as a collection of quite diverse clinical specialties. A thorough knowledge of the processes responsible for the maintenance of health and the development of disease enables a more complete understanding of the role of modern medicine in diagnosis and patient management. Understanding the natural history of diseases allows the determination of prognosis (patient outlook) and may allow the development of strategies for disease screening (checking for the presence of disease at an early stage). The elucidation of molecular mechanisms involved in the development of disease processes has led to an increasing variety of specific therapies that influence defined molecular pathways. The subspecialties within pathology are also clinical specialties in which pathologists are closely involved with patient care.

Cellular pathology and patient management

Cellular pathology (histopathology and cytopathology) is often seen as the 'gold standard' for the diagnosis of many neoplastic and non-neoplastic disease processes. Histological examination of cytology specimens or small tissue biopsies often provides the definitive diagnosis for a patient and, therefore, directs subsequent treatment. Accurate examination of larger tissue fragments or organs removed at surgery is important to ensure that the original diagnosis was correct, to guide further management (i.e. patient treatment) and to determine the patient's prognosis (outlook).

Cellular pathologists work closely with other clinical staff. In the UK, pathologists are members of multidisciplinary teams of healthcare professionals involved in patient care within the modern NHS. Such teams were formed primarily to improve the standard of care for cancer patients, but similar teams are nowadays also responsible for many other diseases. Cancer multidisciplinary teams would include specialist surgeons, physicians, oncologists (cancer doctors who prescribe radiotherapy and chemotherapy), radiologists and cellular pathologists, as well as specialist nurses and palliative care teams. The most common cancers are diagnosed and treated within most hospitals, while patient care for more unusual cancers is now becoming centralized within regional or supraregional centres. This organization ensures that the expertise required for the highest quality of patient care is focused in larger centres where sufficient numbers of patients with rare tumour types are treated. Within each hospital or region, each group of cancer types (e.g. breast cancer, colorectal cancer, urological cancer) possesses its own multidisciplinary team. At the regular (e.g. weekly) meetings between team members, individual patients are discussed to ensure that their diagnosis is accurate and that they are receiving the most appropriate treatment.

Further roles of cellular pathologists
Autopsy work
Cellular pathologists perform postmortem examinations, most commonly for medicolegal reasons at the request of a coroner (or Procurator Fiscal in Scotland) but also if requested by a deceased patient's family or the clinical team caring for the patient (the 'hospital request' autopsy).

The role of a medicolegal postmortem examination is primarily to establish the cause of death and the examination may be followed by an inquest (i.e. an inquiry into the circumstances surrounding the death), which is held by a coroner, especially if the death occurred through unnatural causes (e.g. deaths from accidents or suicide). Pathologists are often asked to attend inquests and give evidence as professional witnesses relating to the medical cause of death. Information from the autopsy may also be important in providing evidence of the identity of the deceased or of the time of death. Specialist forensic pathologists are usually involved in cases where the circumstances raise the possibility of homicide.

Hospital-requested postmortem examinations are performed for a variety of reasons: for example, if the clinical team members believe that they know the cause of death but wish to gain a more complete understanding of a patient's illness. Such examinations may only be performed with written consent from the deceased patient's family.

Important disease processes that are different from or additional to those diagnosed during life are often discovered at postmortem examination, even when the most modern diagnostic tests have been used during the patient's treatment. Therefore, both medicolegal and hospital request postmortem examinations form a very important means of clinical audit (i.e. ensuring that the standard of care received by patients is of the highest quality).

Research
The dual roles of cellular pathology as a basic medical science and a clinical speciality mean that the subject is a cornerstone of medical research. Histological confirmation of a disease process is often an entrance criterion for trials of new treatments while studies of disease development and indicators of prognosis and likely response to novel treatments are often only practically possible using stored tissue samples within cellular pathology laboratories. The expertise of cellular pathologists in microscopic interpretation of tissue alterations in disease is often a key element in successful research.

Quality assurance
It is essential that pathology laboratories provide a consistently high quality of service and mechanisms exist to ensure that this occurs. This process is termed **quality assurance** and may occur as a locally, regionally or nationally organized exercise.

Teaching and training
The dual roles of pathology as a basic medical science and a clinical specialty mean that teaching is an important activity for pathologists. Pathologists within hospitals attached to undergraduate medical schools will usually teach medical students, while many pathology laboratories train the pathologists of the future. In the UK, to become a consultant in cellular pathology requires qualification as a doctor followed by the completion of preregistration house posts. At this stage, young doctors may enter cellular pathology training directly (an increasingly common practice) or first undertake basic training within one or more clinical specialties.

High return facts

1 Cellular and tissue growth is a normal component of normal physiology. Complex intra- and intercellular signalling mechanisms control the rate and extent of growth. Many disease processes are characterized by alterations in the rate and control of cellular and tissue turnover. Defects in these normal control mechanisms may lead to disease states such as neoplasia.

2 There are several ways in which the constituents of the body can alter in size in association with a normal physiological mechanism or as part of a disease process. Cells and tissues may increase in size via hyperplasia or hypertrophy, while a decrease in size occurs via atrophy. Metaplasia is the process whereby differentiated (i.e. mature) cells change from one type to another. Cells die in two major mechanisms: apoptosis and necrosis.

3 Inflammation is a major component of the response to cellular and tissue injury. It is characterized by increased blood flow (redness and warmth: *rubor* and *calor*), swelling (*tumor*) and pain (*dolor*) within the affected area, as well as systemic effects including malaise and pyrexia.

4 Acute inflammation occurs during the early phase of a reaction to cellular/tissue damage. It is characterized histologically by the presence of acute inflammatory cells (neutrophils) within the affected tissue. Acute inflammation may resolve if the underlying stimulus is removed, or it may progress to chronic inflammation.

5 Acute inflammation occurs through the release of inflammatory mediators from damaged tissues and other cells. This leads to a combination of increased vascular permeability and chemotaxis: attraction of inflammatory cells to the area secondary to the release of chemicals from the site of inflammation.

6 Chronic inflammation may occur de novo or develop as a sequel to acute inflammation, especially if the source of cellular/tissue damage persists. It is characterized histologically by the presence of chronic inflammatory cells: lymphocytes, plasma cells and macrophages. Granulomatous inflammation is a special form of chronic inflammation characterized histologically by the presence of granulomas: localized collections of macrophages. Multinucleate giant cells may also be present. Causes of granulomatous inflammation include tuberculosis, fungal infections, tissue reactions to foreign material and specific diseases such as sarcoidosis and Crohn's disease.

7 The resolution of inflammation is associated with organization of the inflammatory reaction: granulation tissue formation and myofibroblast proliferation. This is followed by a variable degree of collagen deposition (fibrous scarring). Collagen deposition is generally more pronounced if the inflammatory process has been prolonged.

8 A range of chemicals that are released from damaged tissues and inflammatory cells orchestrates the inflammatory process (e.g. histamine, prostaglandins, leukotrienes). Protein cascades originating within the plasma are also important in regulating the response to tissue injury (e.g. coagulation, fibrinolytic, complement and kinin cascades).

9 Cells and tissues may be damaged by a range of insults; these may be physical (trauma and extremes of heat), chemical (e.g. acid), neoplastic (e.g. cancers infiltrating adjacent tissue), infective (e.g. bacterial pneumonia), immune (e.g. autoimmune diseases such as rheumatoid arthritis) or iatrogenic (e.g. drugs causing gastric ulceration).

10 There are two major mechanisms by which cells can die. Apoptosis (programmed cell death) is an energy-requiring process leading to death of individual cells, which does not incite an inflammatory reaction. Apoptosis may be physiological or pathological in nature. Necrosis does not require energy, usually affects groups of cells and typically incites an inflammatory reaction—usually acute in nature.

11 Various degenerative processes can occur within cells and tissues as a result of disease states. For example, calcification may occur if the serum calcium concentration is chronically elevated ('metastatic' calcification) or within an abnormal tissue (e.g. a tumour or focus of chronic inflammation; 'dystrophic' calcification). Amyloid is an insoluble protein with a β-pleated sheet structure that is deposited either locally or in a widespread manner in various chronic disease states such as chronic inflammatory conditions (e.g. tuberculosis) or low-grade neoplasms of B-lymphocyte lineage (e.g. lymphoplasmacytic lymphoma). Other forms of degenerative change include glycogen accumulation, hyaline change and myxomatous change.

12 Haemosiderin is an iron-containing pigment that may be deposited in tissues following red cell destruction and haemoglobin breakdown (e.g. after a haemorrhage) or within organs such as the liver in genetic haemochromatosis. Lipofuscin is a wear-and-tear pigment that is deposited in organs such as the heart and liver. Melanin is produced by melanocytes in the skin and is commonly found in tumours showing melanocytic differentiation (e.g. malignant melanoma). Bilirubin is a bile pigment that accumulates in jaundice, either in conjugated or unconjugated form.

13 Shock is a clinical condition characterized by a fast pulse rate (usually > 100 beats/min) and a low blood pressure (systolic blood pressure usually < 100 mmHg). Common types of shock are hypovolaemic (low blood volume, e.g. in haemorrhage), cardiogenic (heart pump failure, e.g. in myocardial infarction) and septic (severe infection). Less common types are anaphylactic (type I hypersensitivity reaction, e.g. peanut allergy) and neurogenic (loss of sympathetic vasomotor tone, e.g. in a spinal cord injury).

14 Tissue injury is usually followed by haemostasis, an inflammatory response and tissue restructuring, with a variable degree of scarring. Factors impairing healing include old age, poor nutritional state, excessive tissue damage, poor apposition of the wound edges (or bony fragments after a fracture), the presence of foreign material, poor blood supply and infection.

15 Vasculitis is inflammation of blood vessel walls. It most commonly occurs as part of an autoimmune disease. Blood vessel wall inflammation may lead to leakage of blood from the vessel or to lumenal thrombosis and, therefore, to tissue ischaemia.

16 The body possesses many mechanisms that aim to protect against potentially injurious agents. These mechanisms may be behavioural, anatomical or immunological in nature.

17 Complex systems exist to protect the body from microorganisms. Some of these systems are innate and have a broad-based action while others are acquired and act more specifically. The functions of the immune system are carried out by immunoreactive cells circulating within the blood and present within tissues, as well as by circulating antibodies.

18 Autoimmune diseases occur when the immune system attacks 'self' cells and tissues; this is referred to as a breakdown of 'immune tolerance'. This leads to inflammation and tissue damage, which may be highly localized (e.g. type 1 diabetes mellitus) or generalized (e.g. systemic lupus erythematosus) in nature.

19 Defects may occur within the immune system. These may be congenital (e.g. severe combined immunodeficiency) or acquired (e.g. reaction to chemotherapy, infection with the human immunodeficiency virus (HIV)) in nature. Such defects may affect a specific component of the immune system or have more widespread effects within several components. Defects usually lead to increased susceptibility to a range of infections.

20 Neoplasia means 'new growth' and indicates the presence of cells or tissues showing evidence of abnormally controlled or disordered growth. Neoplasms comprise cells that show differentiation along one or more pathways of development. Benign neoplasms expand locally but do not invade adjacent tissues or spread to distant sites, while the latter two features are characteristics of malignant neoplasms ('cancers').

21 Genetic and environmental factors influence the development of neoplasia. Most germline (i.e. inherited and present in all cells) genetic influences on neoplasm development are polygenic in nature, while a minority of neoplasms occur in association with a clearly defined inherited defect in a single gene. Neoplasms vary in their relative incidence between populations and different geographical areas, as a result of differences in gene pools and environmental contributors to disease development.

22 Neoplasm development is characterized by the accumulation of genetic defects within the neoplastic cells. In some neoplasms, this sequence is well characterized, while in others specific genetic mutations are found sufficiently commonly that their detection may be used to confirm the diagnosis of tissue type or to help to determine the likely biological behaviour of the neoplasm (i.e. how aggressively the neoplasm is likely to grow).

23 Benign tumours may compress adjacent tissue but do not invade it. Malignant tumours grow locally, infiltrate adjacent tissue and metastasize via lymphatic channels and blood vessels to distant sites.

24 Benign tumours can cause death by compressing vital structures (e.g. within the brainstem) but otherwise generally possess a much better prognosis than malignant tumours. Malignant tumours commonly cause extensive local tissue damage, but tumour metastasis to distant sites is often the key process that causes death in advanced malignancy. Benign and malignant tumours may also produce chemicals such as hormones and, therefore, be associated with clinical symptoms of hormone excess.

25 The clinical and pathological features of neoplasms can indicate whether they are benign or malignant in nature. Histopathological examination of malignant neoplasms is important to determine how aggressively the neoplasm is likely to grow and metastasize. Features such as the tumour type, grade (histological assessment of aggressiveness), size and the presence of lymph node metastases are among the most commonly assessed features used to predict the biological behaviour of malignant neoplasms.

26 Lung cancer is an aggressive neoplasm for which cigarette smoking is the major risk factor. Almost all lung cancers are carcinomas. The neoplasm can invade local structures including the mediastinum and chest wall and commonly metastasizes to distant sites. Many patients present when the disease is at an advanced local stage or with widespread metastases and when surgical removal is not possible.

27 Breast cancer is the second most common malignancy in women (only exceeded by lung cancer in populations where cigarette smoking is common). Almost all breast cancers are carcinomas. These neoplasms most often present as breast masses and invade local structures including the skin and breast wall as well as metastasizing to local lymph nodes and distant sites. While breast cancer is an important cause of mortality among middle-aged and older women, modern advances in therapy have significantly improved the outcome from this disease.

28 Colorectal cancer is one of the three most common cancers in Western populations; it is likely that environmental factors, including the Western diet with low roughage, contribute to this. Almost all colorectal cancers are carcinomas. These neoplasms grow locally and patients may present with rectal bleeding, a change in bowel habit or with acute abdominal symptoms caused by bowel obstruction or perforation. Metastasis to local lymph nodes and distant sites (most commonly the liver) may occur. Surgical removal when the disease is localized to the bowel wall is often associated with a favourable outcome.

29 Prostatic cancer is increasing in incidence among middle-aged and elderly men, although this may partly reflect increased detection of the disease in its early stages in screening programmes. Almost all prostatic cancers are carcinomas. These neoplasms may invade local pelvic structures and metastasize to distant sites, especially bone. While advanced prostatic cancer is commonly fatal, localized disease (most commonly identified by screening) may be curable with prostatectomy. The progression of advanced disease may also be slowed with hormonal therapy.

30 Disease screening means attempting to detect disease processes at an early (asymptomatic) stage when prompt treatment should result in an improved prognosis. Diseases are required to fit various criteria in order to be suitable for screening. UK screening programmes are currently in place for neoplastic diseases such as breast and cervical cancer and for non-neoplastic diseases such as neonatal hypothyroidism and phenylketonuria.

31 The body is particularly susceptible to certain conditions at the extremes of age. Premature babies possess immature body systems and are prone to infections and specific difficulties associated with organs that are not fully developed (e.g. respiratory failure, gut failure). Certain neoplasms occur primarily in childhood (e.g. neuroblastoma, nephroblastoma). Elderly individuals develop wear-and-tear diseases (e.g. osteoarthritis), atherosclerosis-associated conditions (e.g. ischaemic heart disease) and are at increased risk of many neoplasms.

32 Congenital diseases are those that are present at birth. Inherited diseases are those passed on from parents via the transfer of a genetic defect (e.g. familial adenomatous polyposis). Congenital diseases may be inherited from parents but may also occur though chromosomal abnormalities that originate during gametogenesis or fertilization (e.g. Down's syndrome) or 'insults' sustained by the fetus before birth (e.g. congenital infections).

33 Although neoplasm development is commonly associated with genetic abnormalities within the neoplastic tissue, the proportion of neoplasms that occur as a result of a single inherited germline genetic abnormality (i.e. a mutation present within all of the cells making up an individual) is relatively low. Examples include inherited predispositions to breast cancer and colorectal cancer. Although relatively uncommon, these inherited syndromes are important since affected individuals may develop cancer at a young age and sometimes develop multiple cancers. Identification of affected families may allow cancer prevention programmes and/or the detection of cancers at an early stage.

34 Atherosclerosis is a very common disease process occurring within arteries, especially large elastic arteries and their major branches. The earliest lesions comprise 'fatty streaks' within the arterial intima. Established atherosclerotic plaques comprise a 'cap' of fibrous tissue beneath which are pools of fat, foamy macrophages and smooth muscle cells. Dystrophic calcification is common in older lesions. The plaque surface may ulcerate (plaque rupture), leading to a thrombus that coats the plaque.

35 Ischaemic heart disease is the leading cause of death among adults within Western populations. It occurs secondary to narrowing of one or more of the coronary arteries, most commonly as a result of atherosclerotic changes. Ischaemic heart disease commonly results in angina and may lead to myocardial infarction and/or cardiac failure. Sudden death may occur with or without evidence of myocardial infarction.

36 Apart from ischaemic heart disease, atherosclerosis also commonly affects the carotid and intracranial arteries, leading to cerebrovascular disease (e.g. strokes, vascular dementia) while aortic and iliac artery atherosclerosis leads to aortic aneurysm formation and peripheral vascular disease (e.g. intermittent claudication and foot gangrene).

37 Thrombosis occurs after activation of the clotting cascade and is a vital physiological mechanism for limiting blood loss when haemorrhage occurs. Thrombosis occurring as part of a disease process may lead to local vascular occlusion (e.g. coronary artery thrombosis) or to distant vascular occlusion (thromboembolism, e.g. pulmonary thromboembolism secondary to deep vein thrombosis). An embolism occurs when an embolus migrates from one part of the body and causes a blockage of a distant blood vessel; the embolus can be made up of materials other than a thrombus, for example air, amniotic fluid and tumour tissue.

38 The mitral and aortic valves are the valves most commonly affected by degenerative disease in adults. Stenosis or incompetence of these valves may lead to cardiac failure and (apart from mitral stenosis) left ventricular cardiac hypertrophy, while aortic stenosis is a not uncommon cause of sudden death. Rheumatic fever is an important cause of mitral valve stenosis in older patients. Damaged cardiac valves are prone to secondary bacterial infection, which itself can lead to further valvular damage. There are many forms of congenital heart disease resulting in anatomical abnormalities of the heart (e.g. ventricular septal defect, valvular atresia) and associated structures (e.g. patent ductus arteriosus). Congenital heart defects leading to the introduction of systemic venous blood directly into the systemic arterial circulation commonly cause cyanosis.

39 Unusual conditions of the myocardium such as viral myocarditis and cardiomyopathy (e.g. hypertrophic cardiomyopathy) are important causes of sudden death in young adults. Cardiomyopathies may result from a genetic defect or occur secondary to cardiac muscle damage, following, for example, viral myocarditis or chronic excess alcohol consumption.

40 Cardiac failure occurs when the heart is unable to eject blood sufficiently effectively during systole. Common causes of heart failure include ischaemic heart disease, cardiac valvular disease, hypertensive heart disease and chronic lung disease. Less common causes include pericardial constriction and dilated cardiomyopathy. Left ventricular cardiac failure results in pulmonary vascular congestion and oedema. Right ventricular cardiac failure produces a raised jugular venous pressure, hepatic venous congestion and peripheral oedema.

41 Hypertension is common, often asymptomatic and has many causes including stress, obesity, renal artery stenosis and hormonal defects such as Cushing's syndrome and Conn's syndrome. Chronic hypertension is characterized by an imbalance in sodium and water homeostasis. Untreated hypertension can lead to accelerated atherosclerosis and to end-organ damage, including hypertensive nephropathy, hypertensive heart disease and intracerebral haemorrhage.

42 Pneumonia means inflammation within the lung and most commonly occurs as a result of an infection. Many microorganisms may infect lung tissue, but among the most common are viruses and bacteria: the latter resulting in the most common and severe forms of pneumonia. Pneumonia may be acquired within the community or while in hospital and these circumstances are associated with different infective organisms. Pneumonia may primarily involve one pulmonary lobe (lobar pneumonia) or be more widespread and centred on respiratory bronchioles (bronchopneumonia). Bronchopneumonia is a common terminal event in patients with other serious diseases.

43 Tuberculosis affects millions of individuals worldwide and most commonly occurs in developing countries. There is a strong association between tuberculosis and HIV infection, particularly in Africa. Tuberculosis is caused by the *Mycobacterium tuberculosis* bacterium and is classically associated with extensive tissue necrosis and granulomatous inflammation. Infection may be localized (e.g. to the lung) or widespread; the latter is commonly fatal. Treatment usually requires prolonged therapy with multiple special antibiotics.

44 Chronic obstructive pulmonary disease is characterized by the presence of emphysema (lung tissue destruction) and chronic bronchitis (excess bronchial mucus and airway wall thickening) in variable proportions. There is a strong association with cigarette smoking. The disease is chronic, results in an 'obstructive' pulmonary function defect and is often complicated by pulmonary infection. Death eventually occurs through respiratory failure, sepsis or right ventricular cardiac failure.

45 Asthma is a reversible obstructive pulmonary airway defect associated with bronchial smooth muscle hypersensitivity and excess bronchial mucus production. An acute asthma attack is characterized by bronchoconstriction and airway blockage by mucus plugs; this leads to wheezing and in very severe cases respiratory failure (status asthmaticus). Treatment with inhaled bronchodilators (e.g. β_2-adrenoceptor agonists) and anti-inflammatory agents (e.g. inhaled steroids) is effective in the majority of patients.

46 Diseases that make the lung tissue stiffer result in restrictive lung disease: the lungs are unable to expand fully and the total lung capacity is reduced. Conditions most commonly associated with a restrictive lung function defect include fibrosis (e.g. cryptogenic fibrosing alveolitis, asbestosis).

47 Peptic ulcer disease is common in Western populations and involves mucosal ulceration within the stomach and duodenum. *Helicobacter pylori* infection is by far the most common underlying cause. Peptic ulcers cause abdominal pain while complications include gastrointestinal haemorrhage and perforation of the gastric or duodenal wall. Perforation usually causes peritonitis but perforation into the pancreas may cause acute pancreatitis.

48 Malabsorption of nutrients from food may be caused by pancreatic exocrine insufficiency (e.g. chronic pancreatitis) or by a specific or generalized defect within the luminal gastrointestinal tract. Specific defects include pernicious anaemia (damage to the intrinsic factor-producing parietal cells within specialized gastric mucosa) while generalized defects include post-infectious diarrhoea (damage to the small intestinal microvillous brush border).

49 Gallstones are very common. They occur when cholesterol or bile pigments crystallize within concentrated bile and usually form within the gallbladder. Complications include acute and chronic cholecystitis, obstructive jaundice and acute pancreatitis.

50 Acute pancreatitis is a potentially life-threatening condition that most commonly occurs secondary to alcohol abuse and/or gallstones. Chronic pancreatitis is an insidious condition that most commonly develops secondary to chronic alcohol abuse. Both conditions can lead to pancreatic exocrine (and sometimes endocrine) insufficiency.

51 'Primary' type 1 diabetes mellitus occurs secondary to autoimmune destruction of pancreatic insulin-producing beta cells in the islet. Type 1 diabetes develops most commonly in children and young adults as a result of a combination of an inherited genetic predisposition to autoimmune disease plus a triggering factor that may be a viral infection. Type 2 diabetes occurs primarily though increasing resistance of peripheral tissues to insulin and it typically develops in middle-aged and elderly people, where it is closely associated with obesity. Diabetes mellitus may also occur as a secondary phenomenon in conditions such as Cushing's disease or as a side effect of treatments such as steroid therapy.

52 Acute complications of diabetes mellitus include hyperglycaemia with ketoacidosis (type 1 diabetes) or hyperosmolar coma (type 2 diabetes) and hypoglycaemia; hypoglycaemia occurs secondary to therapy (i.e. insulin replacement in type 1 or oral hypoglycaemic agents in type 2). Chronic complications include an increased susceptibility to infections, accelerated atherosclerosis and microvascular angiopathy, leading to retinopathy, for example, and forming a component of diabetic nephropathy.

53 Fatty change is a common liver condition with many causes, including excess alcohol consumption, diabetes mellitus, obesity, drug reactions and various other forms of metabolic disturbance. Cirrhosis is nodular transformation of the liver characterized by hepatocyte regeneration together with bands of fibrous scar tissue. The numerous causes for cirrhosis include chronic alcohol abuse, viral hepatitis and autoimmune conditions (e.g. autoimmune hepatitis, primary biliary cirrhosis).

54 Urinary tract infections are much more common in females than males and usually occur secondary to infection with faecal bacteria such as *Escherichia coli*. Infections commonly involve the bladder (causing cystitis) but may also involve the kidneys (causing pyelonephritis). Predisposing factors include female gender, urinary calculi and urinary stasis. Urinary tract infections are a common cause of septicaemia, especially within the elderly.

55 Glomerulonephritis means inflammation centred on glomeruli; the remainder of the nephron may show secondary changes. Glomerulonephritis may occur as an acute or chronic condition and causes nephritic syndrome (especially in children), nephrotic syndrome and renal failure (acute and chronic). There are multiple causes and several distinct histological subtypes, each with a different clinical outcome.

56 Raised intracranial pressure may occur secondary to intracranial haemorrhage (usually acute onset) or as a result of a space-occupying lesion such as a neoplasm (usually gradual onset). Early effects include cranial nerve compression (e.g. third nerve compression leading to pupillary dilatation) while later effects include herniation of brain tissue through an anatomical aperture (e.g. the foramen magnum), which when severe may lead to brainstem compression and death.

57 Strokes present clinically as sudden neurological defects and may be caused by intracranial haemorrhage (e.g. subarachnoid or intracranial haemorrhage) or cerebral infarction (usually secondary to thrombotic or embolic occlusion of a carotid or intracranial artery). Strokes may lead to death or permanent severe neurological defects, but modern therapies can result in remarkable clinical recovery.

58 Dementia is a progressive global decline in intellectual capacity that occurs with increasing frequency with advancing age. The two most commonly encountered forms are Alzheimer's disease (sometimes familial) and vascular (multi-infarct) dementia. Less common dementias are Huntington's disease (an inherited condition) and Pick's disease.

59 Osteoporosis is loss of bone matrix (density) and most commonly occurs in postmenopausal women; hormone replacement therapy is an important prophylaxis against its development. Osteomalacia is loss of bone mineralization and occurs because of poor dietary vitamin D intake or defects in vitamin D and calcium metabolism (e.g. chronic renal failure). Osteoporosis and osteomalacia predispose to fractures, especially of the hip, wrist and thoracolumbar spine.

60 Osteoarthritis is a wear-and-tear condition most commonly affecting major weight-bearing joints and characterized by erosion of articular cartilage and osteophyte formation. Predisposing factors include 'excess' physical activity (e.g. sports people) and prior damage to the joint or associated bones; both result in abnormal joint stresses. Rheumatoid arthritis is a multisystem disorder comprising a symmetrical inflammatory polyarthritis together with extra-articular manifestations including pulmonary fibrosis and subcutaneous nodules.

61 Endocrine hormones are key factors in the regulation of metabolism, and the correct regulation of their production is essential. Excess endocrine hormone production results in conditions such as Cushing's syndrome (excess glucocorticosteroids), Conn's syndrome (excess mineralocorticoids), Graves' disease (excess thyroid hormone) and acromegaly (excess growth hormone). Insufficient endocrine hormone production results in conditions such as Addison's disease (insufficient corticosteroids) and hypothyroidism.

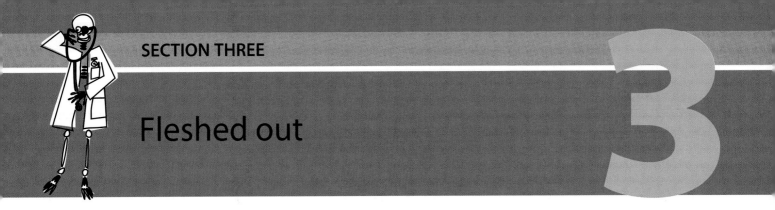

Fleshed out

Section three expands on each of the high return facts within an easy-to-read double page spread. Where possible, tables and illustrations are used to impart information and aid the understanding of each key disease process. The chapters are grouped together in the following way: key concepts and processes within pathology (1–16), basic immunology (17–19), neoplasia (20–29), screening (30), age-related, congenital and inherited diseases (31–33), cardiovascular disease (34–41), respiratory disease (42–46), gastrointestinal disease and diabetes (47–53), urinary tract disease (54 and 55), nervous system disease (56–58), musculoskeletal disease (59 and 60) and endocrine disease (61).

1. Growth and differentiation

Questions
- How is the growth and maturation of cells and tissues controlled?
- What is the cell cycle?

The characteristics of a tissue depend on the balance between the rate at which cells proliferate, the type of differentiation they exhibit and the rate at which they die. Except for the germ cells of the ovary and testis, which divide by meiosis, the cells of the human body proliferate by mitotic division, in which a full copy of the genome is distributed into each of the two daughter cells. Apoptosis is programmed cell death; it is involved in many different physiological and pathological processes (Ch. 10).

If multicellular organisms are to grow and develop successfully, the proliferation, differentiation and death of cells must be tightly controlled. Evolution has provided the human body with an extremely complex network of interconnecting control systems, and these systems are involved in almost all pathological processes.

Control of proliferation, differentiation and apoptosis

The principal way in which cells communicate with their surroundings is by receptors. The binding site of a receptor is capable of binding in a highly specific way to another molecule (or part of a molecule) called a **ligand**. When a receptor binds to its ligand, the tertiary structure of the receptor changes. This change in structure is associated with the initiation of biochemical events inside the cell that act to control its metabolism or the expression of genes. An example is the interaction between an integrin receptor and fibronectin, which is a way in which cells interact with the extracellular matrix (Fig. 3.1.1). The integrins are a member of the family of transmembrane receptors called **cell adhesion molecules.** Fibronectin is an extracellular matrix protein that binds to collagen and other matrix molecules. It also binds to, and acts as a ligand for, integrin. When this interaction occurs, the conformational change in the intracellular integrin domain promotes interaction between the integrin molecule and components of the cytoskeleton and also initiates the activation of second messengers that can have a variety of effects, including control of progression through the cell cycle.

The binding between receptor and ligand is highly specific. It has been likened to the fit between a lock and a key. An alternative analogy is that of a hand in a glove, since complex biochemical molecules come in left-handed and right-handed forms (stereoisomerism).

Control systems can be divided into three main types.

Soluble mediators. Soluble mediators act as ligands for specific receptors. The effects can be categorized as **autocrine** (the ligand acts on the cell that produced it), **paracrine** (it acts on adjacent cells), **endocrine** (it circulates through the bloodstream to the target cells), and **synaptic** (it is secreted into the synaptic cleft by a nerve cell as a result of depolarization). The term 'growth factor' is often applied to substances with autocrine and paracrine effects, while the term 'hormone' is often used for endocrine substances. However, this distinction is not clear-cut and many substances can have autocrine, paracrine, endocrine and even synaptic effects depending on the circumstances. Furthermore, growth factors can have effects on differentiation and apoptosis as well as on cell proliferation.

Cell–cell interactions. Cells can interact directly with each other via receptors expressed on the cell membranes. Molecules expressed on the target cells act as ligands in these circumstances.

Cell–matrix interactions. The intercellular matrix is a dynamic complex of many different substances that not only provides mechanical support for tissues but also promotes and maintains differentiation of epithelia and regulates cell multiplication (Fig. 3.1.1).

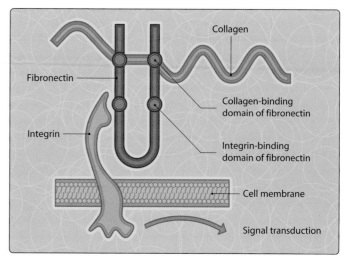

Fig. 3.1.1 The integrins are a group of transmembrane receptors important in transmitting growth and differentiation signals from the extracellular matrix. Here, integrin binds fibronectin, a matrix molecule that can bind to both collagen and integrin. The resulting conformational change in integrin activates intracellular signal transduction.

Cell cycle

In order to divide, a cell has to go through the **cell cycle** (Fig. 3.1.2). During gap phase 1 (G_1), the cell prepares to replicate its DNA. This process occurs during synthesis (S) phase, and the total amount of DNA in the cell doubles as this happens. After the genome has been replicated, the cell prepares to divide during gap phase 2 (G_2). Mitosis, or M phase, follows, and two daughter cells are produced.

The daughter cells can continue in the cell cycle and divide again. Alternatively, they can enter a condition known as G_0, which could be associated with differentiation of the cell. While in G_0, the cell is not actively dividing. However, if suitably stimulated, it can reenter the cell cycle and start to replicate again. A further option for the daughter cells is to undergo terminal differentiation; such cells lose the ability to undergo mitosis and cannot reenter the cell cycle.

The stem cell concept

Stem cells are capable of repeated division and, therefore, represent the source of the various cells that make up the body. Stem cells can exhibit asymmetrical division, in which one daughter cell differentiates while the other remains in the cell cycle, or symmetrical division, in which both daughter cells remain in the cell cycle (Fig. 3.3.3). Tissues in which cells are constantly being lost require constantly active stem cells to replace the lost cells. Examples of such tissues (sometimes called labile tissues) are the skin and the epithelia lining the gastrointestinal tract.

If cells that are not stem cells are grown in tissue culture and stimulated to divide, the number of divisions is limited. For example, fibroblasts in vitro will undergo perhaps 50 or 60 divisions at most; no amount of stimulation will induce further division. This phenomenon is controlled by **telomeres**, which are noncoding sequences of repeating base-pairs at the end of each chromosome. With each mitosis, a short segment of each telomere is lost. When the telomeres become too short, mitosis cannot occur. Thus, the telomeres act as a kind of clock, counting down the number of permitted cell divisions. However, stem cells are capable of dividing indefinitely because they possess **telomerase**, an enzyme that reconstitutes the telomeres at each cell division, thus maintaining their length. Telomerase activity is also expressed in most neoplasms and represents one way in which neoplasms escape from the normal control of cell growth.

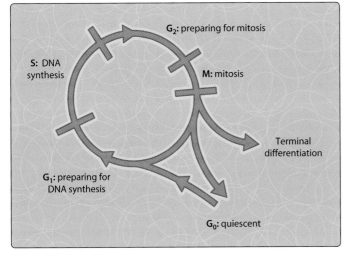

Fig. 3.1.2 The cell cycle.

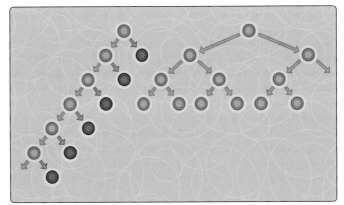

Fig. 3.1.3 Asymmetrical and symmetrical stem cell division. When a stem cell (blue) divides, one of the daughter cells can become terminally differentiated (red), as shown on the left. This is asymmetrical stem cell division. Alternatively, both daughter cells can remain in the cell cycle as shown on the right. This is symmetrical stem cell division.

2. Patterns of growth in health and disease

Questions
- What are the mechanisms by which cells die?
- How do cells and tissues change in life?

The growth of cells and tissues is an essential normal process. Cells and tissues possess a defined lifespan and the continued survival of the whole individual is dependent upon the successful removal and replacement of effete (i.e. worn out) cells with new counterparts. Tissues also require the capacity to change their size in response to a wide range of physiological stimuli:

- normal development from conception to adulthood
- increase in uterine mass during pregnancy
- increase in breast tissue mass prior to breastfeeding
- increase in skeletal muscle mass in athletes
- increase in kidney size after contralateral nephrectomy
- decrease in thymic gland mass during childhood
- decrease in skeletal muscle mass owing to weightlessness or immobilization
- decrease in uterine mass at the menopause.

Changes to the normal mechanisms governing tissue kinetics can result in abnormal tissue growth and the development of neoplasia (Chs 20–25) as well as many aspects of non-neoplastic disease (e.g. an abnormally enlarged heart).

Normal cellular kinetics

Almost all tissues undergo a normal physiological process of cellular 'management' that involves the removal of effete or damaged cells and their replacement by new mature cells. The rate of cellular turnover is extremely variable between tissues. Tissues possessing the highest rates of turnover include the bone marrow and the epithelial cells lining the gastrointestinal tract. These tissues show the highest rates of cell division and are, therefore, the most susceptible to 'collateral' damage by chemotherapeutic treatments that inhibit cell division. Microscopic examination of biopsy samples from these tissues reveals easily identifiable evidence of cell division (i.e. mitotic figures) in normal situations. Many other tissues show a much lower rate of cell turnover but retain the ability to increase in size by cell division when required. The best example of this is the liver, which can return to a normal size even after partial surgical hepatectomy. Some mature tissues possess little or no capacity for cell division. The prime example is central nervous tissue, which also is essentially made up of cells with no extracellular connective tissue matrix. These combined features lead to the limited capacity for recovery from major insults such as extensive cerebral infarction,

which is established by detecting a cystic space within the brain. Another example is the heart, with myocardial cell death (e.g. in infarction) leading to healing by fibrous scar tissue formation rather than complete repair via cardiac myocyte cell division. This means that extensive myocardial infarction commonly interferes significantly with the contractile ability of the left ventricle and, therefore, predisposes to heart failure.

Key mechanisms in cell turnover

Two major mechanisms exist by which cells can 'die' and several mechanisms exist by which tissues and whole organs may increase or reduce in size:

- cell death
  - necrosis
  - apoptosis
- change in size
  - hyperplasia
  - hypertrophy
  - atrophy.

Necrosis

Necrosis describes the morphological (i.e. visible) appearances of cells and tissues after their death via a non-programmed mechanism. Necrosis usually affects groups of cells or even whole organs and characteristically occurs in disease states in which the cells or tissues have been subjected to a major insult (Chs 9 and 10). Necrosis is not, therefore, an event that is orchestrated by individual cells and does not require energy. Necrosis is characteristically associated with an inflammatory infiltrate: typically neutrophils in the early phase of the process.

Apoptosis

Apoptosis describes cell death that occurs as a preprogrammed event initiated within the cells themselves; classically, it affects individual cells but it may also involve groups of cells. The process is energy dependent and may occur as a normal physiological event or as a response to disease states. Examples include

- removal of webs between fingers during prenatal development (failure of apoptosis may result in persistently webbed fingers in neonates)
- removal of autoreactive T-lymphocytes from circulation (loss of this mechanism may contribute to the development of autoimmune disease)
- reduction of breast tissue mass after cessation of breastfeeding
- removal of effete white blood cells from circulation

- loss of 'old' epithelial cells lining gastrointestinal tract during normal cell turnover
- loss of beta cells in pancreatic islets, leading to diabetes mellitus
- reduction of neoplastic tissue mass as a result of hormonal, radio- or chemotherapy.

Failure of apoptosis may lead to congenital abnormalities or the development of neoplasia.

Mechanisms of changing size in tissues or organs

Tissues and organs may increase in size predominantly through hyperplasia or hypertrophy or through a combination of these processes (Table 3.2.1).

Hyperplasia

Hyperplasia describes an increase in the size of a tissue or entire organ as a result of an increase in the *number* of its constituent cells. The capacity for cell division and, therefore, an increase in size by this mechanism is extremely variable between tissues. Tissues such as the endometrium, breast and prostate possess the ability to increase in size by hyperplasia while cardiac muscle possesses very limited capacity for cell division (see below). Hyperplasia most commonly occurs as a result of changes in circulating hormone levels.

Hypertrophy

Hypertrophy describes an increase in the size of a tissue or entire organ as a result of an increase in *size* of its individual constituent cells. An increase in heart size (in response, for example, to aortic valve stenosis or chronic systemic hypertension) occurs almost entirely through hypertrophy of cardiac myocytes (Fig. 3.2.1). Hypertrophy most commonly is a consequence of a change in local conditions affecting the tissue/organ (e.g. increased cardiac myocyte strain in hypertension or increased skeletal muscle strain in athletes).

Atrophy

Atrophy is the term used to describe a decrease in the size of a tissue or entire organ as a result of a decrease in the number *or* size of its constituent cells (Table 3.2.1). Atrophy may occur secondary to changes in circulating hormone levels (e.g. uterine atrophy at the menopause) or through a reduction in use of the tissue/organ (e.g. disuse skeletal muscle atrophy secondary to immobilization of a broken bone).

Metaplasia

Sometimes, cells in injured tissue change to another type that is better able to withstand the cause of the injury. For example, chronic irritation from tobacco smoke can cause the respiratory mucosa of the airways to transform into stratified squamous mucosa. The replacement of one tissue by another in this way is called metaplasia. Two examples of metaplasia in the bladder are shown in Fig. 3.2.2.

Table 3.2.1 MECHANISMS OF ALTERATION IN TISSUE SIZE

Mechanism	Clinical example
Hyperplasia	Increase in breast tissue mass during breastfeeding Increase in thyroid gland mass in Graves' disease
Hypertrophy	Increase in left ventricle cardiac muscle mass in hypertension Increase in skeletal muscle mass in athletes
Atrophy	Decrease in uterine mass at the menopause Decrease in skeletal muscle mass after immobilization

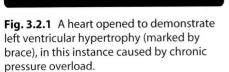

Fig. 3.2.1 A heart opened to demonstrate left ventricular hypertrophy (marked by brace), in this instance caused by chronic pressure overload.

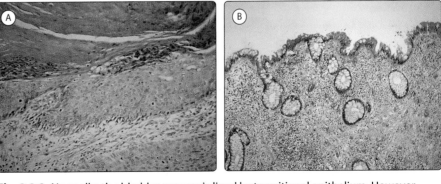

Fig. 3.2.2 Normally, the bladder mucosa is lined by transitional epithelium. However, long-standing chronic inflammation can cause the mucosa to change to another type (i.e. to become metaplastic). These sections from a chronically inflamed bladder show keratinizing squamous metaplasia (A) and glandular metaplasia (B).

3. Inflammation: general principles

Questions
- What is inflammation?
- What is phagocytosis and how does it occur?
- What are the systemic effects of an inflammatory response?

Inflammation is the complex coordinated response by vascularized tissue to injury or microorganisms, mediated by:

- the cells and vessels of the tissue
- cells derived from bone marrow precursors: white blood cells and platelets
- circulating proteins, including clotting factors, fibrinolytic factors, complement and antibodies.

The word inflammation derives from the Latin for burning. Celsus, the Roman physician, in the first century AD described the four **cardinal signs**: *calor* (heat), *rubor* (redness), *dolor* (pain) and *tumor* (swelling). These derive from a series of events.

1. Dilation of small blood vessels and increased local blood flow will produce redness and heat
2. Exudation of fluid into the extravascular space causes swelling and pain
3. Release of substances such as bradykinin, prostaglandins and serotonin produces pain and leads to systemic effects
4. Systemic response of fever is initiated by cytokines that are released into the circulation (a manifestation of calor).

The suffix *-itis* signifies inflammation: appendicitis is inflammation of the appendix and arthritis that of joints.

Through inflammation, evolution has equipped the body with a powerful response to tissue damage and to invasion by microorganisms. However, it is a two-edged sword: it is the inflammatory processes themselves, rather than the factors that elicited the inflammation, that are responsible for the clinical features of many diseases. Furthermore, the inflammatory response may be mounted in inappropriate circumstances, for example in autoimmune diseases. Indeed, the potential for inflammation to harm is such that it needs to be tightly controlled by a large number of chemical mediators that interact with cells and with each other in complex interconnected ways (see Ch. 8).

Inflammation is divided into two types: **acute** and **chronic**. It is the time-scale that defines these two terms; acute inflammation lasts hours or days, while chronic inflammation lasts more than a few days and continues as long as the injurious agent persists. These two responses have many things in common but are characterized by different cell types and processes.

Phagocytosis and inflammation

Phagocytosis (Greek for eating and cell) is the process by which a cell engulfs and digests an extracellular particle. Although a number of different cells can exhibit phagocytosis under certain circumstances, two types are specifically adapted to phagocytic functions: **neutrophils** and **macrophages**. These are sometimes called professional phagocytes. They have important roles in the inflammatory response.

Monocytes (macrophage precursors) and neutrophils are produced in the bone marrow and circulate in the blood. At sites of inflammation, they leave the circulation and migrate to the damaged tissues by amoeboid motion. This same amoeboid ability allows the phagocyte to ingest particles such as bacteria and then digest them within a vacuole (Fig. 3.3.1). The digestive enzymes and free radicals (Fig. 3.3.2) may be released into the extracellular space rather than the phagolysosome, especially if the particle is too large to ingest; this can result in severe tissue damage via oxidation of proteins, lipids and DNA. Cells can be protected from damage by enzymes such as catalase, which promotes the breakdown of hydrogen peroxide, and antioxidants such as vitamins C and E, which free radicals convert to less-reactive derivatives. These defences are useful not only in limiting tissue damage from free radicals released in inflammatory processes but also in scavenging free radicals produced in normal cellular metabolism, ionizing radiation and chemical pollutants. Neutrophils and macrophages can act independently of the immune system and are, therefore, part of innate immunity. However, their function is greatly enhanced by the immune system.

T-cell activation. Macrophages and neutrophils are activated by cytokines produced by T-cells. Activated cells show increased phagocytic activity and increased production of bactericidal substances.

Opsonization. Phagocytes have transmembrane receptors for the Fc portion of immunoglobulin and complement component C3b. When immunoglobulin and C3b become attached to bacteria, they promote the ability of phagocytes to attach to them. This process is called opsonization (from the Greek, 'to prepare for the table') and the immunoglobulin and complement are called **opsonins**.

Systemic effects of inflammation

In addition to their local effects, acute and chronic inflammation also have important systemic effects. These are mediated by cytokines, especially tumour necrosis factor (TNF) alpha and interleukin (IL)-1, which circulate around the body and have endocrine effects on the organs.

The first step is attachment: the particle (in this case a bacterium) binds to receptors on the surface of the phagocyte

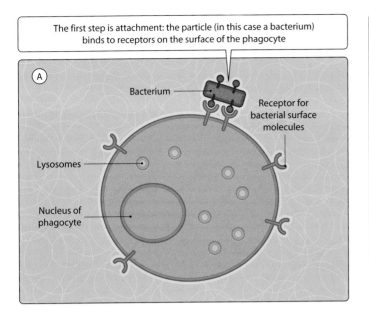

1. Oxygen-independent mechanisms.
These are derived from the lysosome, and include digestive enzymes and substances with specific antimicrobial properties (e.g. the defensins, which form holes in bacterial membranes, and lactoferrin, which chelates the iron required for microbial growth)

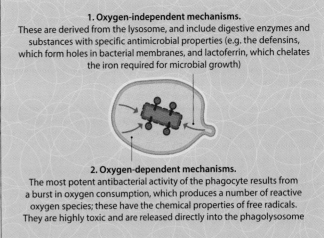

2. Oxygen-dependent mechanisms.
The most potent antibacterial activity of the phagocyte results from a burst in oxygen consumption, which produces a number of reactive oxygen species; these have the chemical properties of free radicals. They are highly toxic and are released directly into the phagolysosome

Fig. 3.3.2 Ingested particles are killed and digested by two types of mechanism.

Pyrexia. The thermoregulatory set-point of the hypothalamus is raised, resulting in a rise in body temperature (fever or pyrexia). This process is often accompanied by constitutional symptoms such as malaise, loss of appetite (anorexia) and nausea. There is also the risk that fever in infants and young children may be associated with fits. Although fever is often treated to improve the general sense of well-being of the patient and, in the case of the young, to reduce the risk of fitting, there is good evidence that fever is an adaptive response to the presence of inflammation since experiments have shown animals are less able to ward off infections if they are prevented from raising their body temperature.

Leukocytosis. White cells are released from the bone marrow and the numbers of circulating white cells increase. The predominant type of cell may act as a diagnostic clue to the cause of the inflammation. For example, a neutrophilia is seen in pyogenic infections, a lymphocytosis is seen in viral infections, and increased eosinophils are seen in allergic reactions and parasitic infestations. When neutrophils are released from the bone marrow in response to cytokine stimulation, the proportion of less-mature forms in the blood increases; haematologists describe this as a 'shift to the left' in neutrophil morphology.

Acute phase protein response. These proteins are mostly derived from the liver. Examples are C-reactive protein (CRP), serum amyloid-A protein (SAA) and fibrinogen. Their serum concentration rises in response to inflammation with a variety of effects. For example, CRP and SAA bind to bacterial cell walls and may act as opsonins. Their presence in the plasma increases the rate at which red cells settle out of a column of blood; this is the basis of the erythrocyte sedimentation rate (ESR) test, which has largely been superseded in clinical practice by measurement of CRP.

Weight loss. The combination of anorexia and increased metabolic activity results in negative nitrogen balance.

In step 2, engulfment, pseudopodia ('false feet') extend around the particle, eventually fusing over the top to form a phagocytic vacuole or phagosome

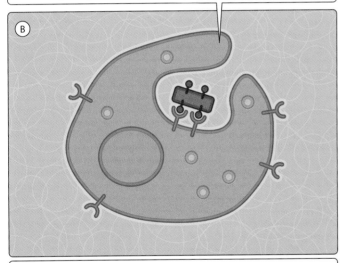

In step 3, intracellular killing, lysosomes fuse to the phagosome, releasing their digestive enzymes into it. This process results in a phagolysosome, within which the particle is destroyed

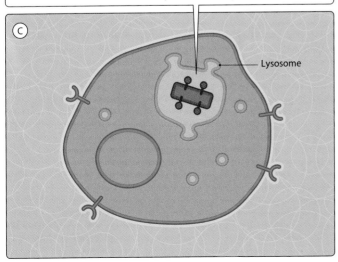

Fig. 3.3.1 Phagocytosis.

4. Acute inflammation: morphology and consequences

Questions
■ What is acute inflammation?
■ How may acute inflammation be manifest in a clinical setting?
■ What are the sequelae of acute inflammation?

A number of morphological patterns of acute inflammation occur depending on the anatomical structures involved, and many descriptive terms have been coined for them.

Morphological appearance

Suppurative (purulent) inflammation

The terms suppurative and purulent imply the production of **pus**, which consists of dead and dying neutrophils, liquefied necrotic tissue and infecting microorganisms. Pus is sticky fluid, typically yellow or grey in colour, although haemorrhage may turn it red or brown. Certain bacteria such as *Staphylococcus aureus* are particularly associated with the production of pus and are, therefore, termed **pyogenic**. Pus is classically described as having a solid component (the neutrophils, necrotic debris and organisms) and a liquid component (the inflammatory exudate and dissolved substances, including nucleic acids, which give pus its sticky characteristics).

Abscesses, sinuses and fistulae

An **abscess** (Fig. 3.4.1) is a collection of pus within tissue. If it persists, it becomes walled off by a surrounding rim of granulation tissue. Sometimes, an abscess will spontaneously discharge via the skin or into a body cavity; it is said to 'point' as it erodes towards the surface of the tissue. When it has burst and discharged its contents, it may be obliterated by granulation tissue and healing will occur by fibrosis. Alternatively, the route along which the pus was discharged may persist as a **sinus tract**, which is defined as a connection between the tissue and a surface (epidermal or epithelial); the tract may be lined by granulation tissue and/or by epithelium derived from the surface. For example, osteomyelitis is often complicated by chronic sinuses connecting the infected bone to the surface of the skin, allowing pus from the site of inflammation to drain. Sometimes, an analogous process will produce a **fistula**, which is an abnormal connection between two epithelial surfaces or an epithelial surface and the skin. For example, a segment of ileum that is inflamed in Crohn's disease may become adherent to the bladder, and if the inflammation spreads into the bladder wall a tract connecting the ileum and the bladder (an ileovesical fistula) may form. A similar process can produce fistulae between the ileum and another segment of bowel, the vagina or the skin. If

a hollow organ (e.g. gallbladder or appendix) or anatomical space (e.g. pleural cavity) fills with pus, the term **empyema** may be used.

Abscesses and other collections of pus can be difficult to treat, since antibiotics may penetrate poorly into the pus-filled cavity. It is for this reason that surgical drainage is usually indicated for a collection of pus.

Inflammation of serous membranes

Acute inflammation of serosal surfaces (pericardium, pleura, peritoneum) is associated with a fibrinogen-rich exudate. The fibrinogen is converted into fibrin, resulting in a roughening of the serosal surface, which is also congested because of dilatation of vessels. The descriptive term for this appearance is **fibrinous inflammation**. A classical example of this phenomenon is 'bread and butter pericarditis', in which acute inflammation of the pericardium causes a fibrinous exudate that resembles the irregular buttery surface that would be observed if a buttered sandwich was pulled apart. If large numbers of neutrophils impart a pus-like appearance to the exudate, the terms **seropurulent exudate** or **fibrinopurulent exudate** may be used.

Inflammation of mucous membranes

The early stages of mucous membrane inflammation produce **catarrhal inflammation**, for example the inflammation seen in the upper respiratory tract as a result of the common cold. Vasodilation and oedema produce reddening and swelling of the mucosa, and the mucus cells secrete large quantities of thin, irritant mucus. If bacterial infection is a component of the disease process, the mucous discharge becomes purulent, producing a **mucopurulent exudate**. In severe bacterial acute inflammation of mucosal surfaces, a collection of neutrophils, dead epithelial cells, fibrin, mucus and infecting organisms collects on the luminal surface. This collection has a membranous appearance and the terms **membranous** or **pseudomembranous inflammation** may be used. (Pseudomembranous is more accurate, because

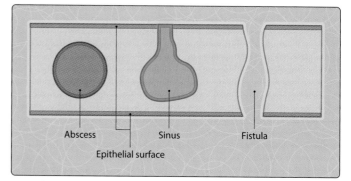

Fig. 3.4.1 Abscess, sinus and fistula.

the slough-like mixture is not a true membrane.) Examples are pseudomembranous colitis in *Clostridium difficile* infection and diphtheria, both of which are characterized by a pale grey or yellow pseudomembrane covering the inflamed mucosa.

Haemorrhagic inflammation

Acute inflammation associated with marked haemorrhage is called haemorrhagic inflammation. A good example is haemorrhagic pancreatitis, in which proteolytic destruction of vessels causes widespread haemorrhage into the pancreatic parenchyma.

Gangrenous (necrotizing) inflammation

As discussed in Ch. 10, the term gangrene generally implies infected necrotic tissue. For example, acute appendicitis can be associated with marked vascular congestion and oedema such that the blood flow becomes inadequate and necrosis occurs. The bowel bacteria multiply in the dead tissue and the resulting putrefaction together with necrosis can be described as gangrenous, or necrotizing, acute appendicitis.

Consequences and sequelae of acute inflammation

Acute inflammation has a number of beneficial effects that represent an effective response to many different types of injury (Fig. 3.4.2). However, it can also have harmful effects:

- normal tissues may be damaged by digestive enzymes released from inflammatory cells
- the tissue swelling can compress blood vessels and cause ischaemia, as in gangrenous appendicitis (see above)
- the tissue swelling can cause obstruction (e.g. the enlarged epiglottis in childhood acute epiglottitis can obstruct the larynx, causing asphyxia)
- the response may be inappropriate, that is, out of proportion to any threat posed by the initiating antigen, such as in type I hypersensitivity reactions
- any resulting scar can have adverse effects (Ch. 7).

The sequelae of acute inflammation depend on the tissue involved, the extent of tissue destruction and the cause of the injury. The possibilities are:

Resolution. The complete restoration of normal structure and function can occur if the tissue is capable of mitotic activity to repopulate the areas of cell loss and if the degree of tissue damage is not too severe. In particular, the preservation of the basement membranes promotes healing by resolution because the cells have a normal matrix on which to grow.

Organization and scarring. If resolution is not possible, granulation tissue forms and ultimately produces a fibrous scar.

Chronic inflammation. If the injurious agent is not rapidly removed, the inflammatory process persists and chronic inflammation develops. For example, if an abscess is not drained it becomes a chronic abscess surrounded by chronically inflamed granulation tissue that gradually organizes the pus to create a fibrous scar. Another example occurs in a gallbladder with gallstones, where the initial acute inflammatory response is converted to chronic inflammation because the gallstones remain within the lumen of the organ.

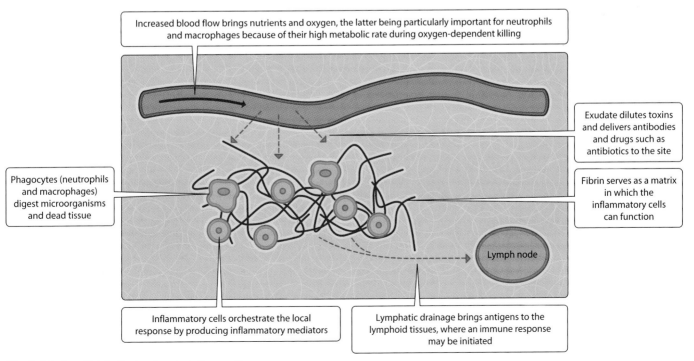

Increased blood flow brings nutrients and oxygen, the latter being particularly important for neutrophils and macrophages because of their high metabolic rate during oxygen-dependent killing

Phagocytes (neutrophils and macrophages) digest microorganisms and dead tissue

Exudate dilutes toxins and delivers antibodies and drugs such as antibiotics to the site

Fibrin serves as a matrix in which the inflammatory cells can function

Lymph node

Inflammatory cells orchestrate the local response by producing inflammatory mediators

Lymphatic drainage brings antigens to the lymphoid tissues, where an immune response may be initiated

Fig. 3.4.2 Beneficial effects of acute inflammation.

5. Acute inflammation: mechanisms

Questions
- What are the cellular changes that occur during acute inflammation?
- What are the functions of the major cell types that are recruited during acute inflammation?

Acute inflammation is the initial reaction of vascularized tissue to an injury. Causes include physical or chemical aetiologies (e.g. trauma, heat cold, radiation, toxins, corrosives), microorganisms or their toxins, infarction and hypersensitivity reactions. The events in acute inflammation are complex and only partially understood. For ease of description, they can be divided into vascular and cellular components (Fig. 3.5.1).

Vascular events

The initial events are active hyperaemia (an increase in blood flow owing to relaxation of precapillary sphincters) and an increase in permeability of the capillaries to plasma proteins, allowing these to leak into the extravascular space. In normal tissues, fluid is forced out at the arterial end of the capillary bed by hydrostatic pressure, but most is reabsorbed at the venous end where the hydrostatic pressure is lower because then the colloid osmotic (or oncotic) pressure gradient exceeds the hydrostatic pressure gradient. Any excess tissue fluid is taken up by the lymphatics. In inflammation,

the colloid osmotic pressure of the blood is reduced because plasma proteins have exuded into the interstitial matrix (Fig. 3.5.2). It appears that plasma proteins can escape by one of two mechanisms:
- as part of the acute inflammatory response, transient gaps appear in the endothelium of venules and small veins because the endothelial cells (which have contractile proteins such as actin in their cytoplasm) contract
- direct damage to the endothelium by physical agents (chemicals, toxins) allows leakage.

Any vessel can be affected by direct damage, whereas transient gaps are confined to venules and small veins. The overall result is both increased hydrostatic pressure, owing to dilatation of precapillary sphincters, and decreased colloid osmotic pressure of the plasma. Consequently, much more fluid leaves the vessels than returns to them and a protein-rich exudate accumulates in the tissues.

The exudate contains proteins that are important in the immune response, and coagulation factors such as fibrinogen (Fig. 3.5.2). The latter promotes the deposition of fibrin, as seen, for example, in the alveolar spaces in pneumonia or the fibrinous exudate on the serosal surfaces of acutely inflamed organs. The continual drainage of tissue fluid by lymphatics ensures that the exudate in the area of inflammation is continually renewed. Furthermore, the lymphatic vessels carry antigens to lymph nodes, where lymphocytes can recognize the antigens and mount an immune response. Fluid loss from plasma increases blood viscosity and slows blood flow; this is the first stage in the emigration of white blood cells into the extravascular space.

Cellular events
Neutrophils
Acute inflammation is characterized by accumulation of neutrophil polymorphonuclear leukocytes (**neutrophils**) in tissues. Their presence in a histological section is the principal way in which histopathologists recognize acute inflammation, and often neutrophils are referred to as the 'acute inflammatory cells'. Neutrophils have a lifespan of only 1–3 days and leave the bloodstream principally from venules. In normal venules, flow dynamics confines cells to the central (axial) part of the lumen, blood immediately adjacent to the endothelium being free of cells. In inflamed tissues, increased plasma viscosity and slowing of flow alters this distribution with a number of consequences.

1. **Margination.** Blood cells flow adjacent to the endothelium, facilitating neutrophil contact with it.
2. **Adhesion (pavementing).** Neutrophils touching the endothelium adhere through bonding between adhesion molecules

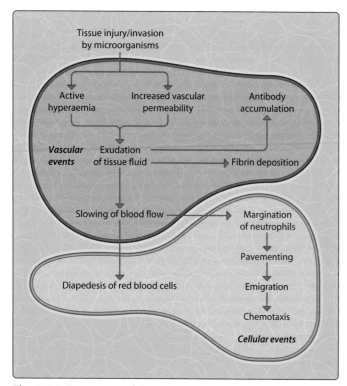

Fig. 3.5.1 A summary of the main events in acute inflammation.

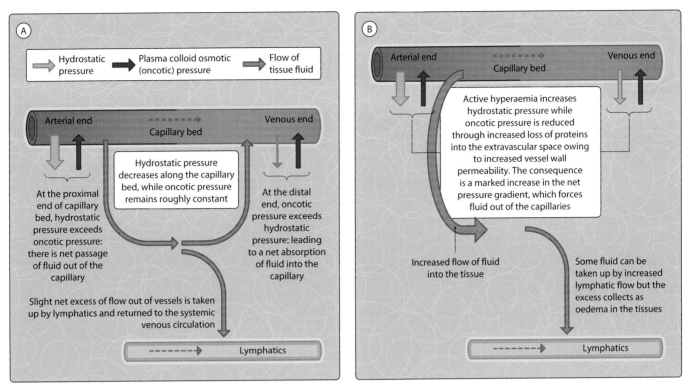

Fig. 3.5.2 Fluid movement in and out of tissues. (A) Normal movement; (B) movement in inflamed tissue.

and their ligands, which are present as transmembrane molecules in both the neutrophils and the endothelial cells. Normally, these adhesion molecules are expressed in small amounts and neutrophils that happen to touch the endothelium do not stick. Inflammation increases the expression (upregulation) of adhesion molecules so that the neutrophils start to adhere to the endothelial surface and roll along it. The selectins are an example of receptors and ligands involved in this phase. After the rolling phase, neutrophils adhere more firmly and come to rest on the endothelial surface.

3. **Emigration (transmigration).** Crawling like an amoeba, the neutrophils leave the blood vessel by squeezing between the endothelial cells.

4. **Chemotaxis.** Neutrophils exhibit chemotaxis (i.e. move along a concentration gradient) and are attracted to sites of injury. Examples of substances chemotactic for neutrophils are some complement components and cytokines. The amoeboid movement of neutrophils depends on complex interactions between the cell and the surrounding matrix.

In severe inflammation, red cells are often observed in the tissues. They have left the bloodstream passively under hydrostatic pressure pushing them through damaged vessel walls. This passive movement of red cells into the tissues is **diapedesis**, and it implies significant damage to the blood vessels. If large numbers of red cells accumulate in inflamed tissues, the iron in their haemoglobin can form haemosiderin aggregates in the macrophages that break down the red cells (Ch. 12).

The principal function of neutrophils is the elimination of the injurious agent by degradative enzymes. This process normally occurs inside the cell following phagocytosis of the offending particle, e.g. a bacterium.

Mast cells

Mast cells store inflammatory mediators such as histamine in their cytoplasmic granules. They can be prompted to degranulate (i.e. release the granule contents into the surrounding tissue) by:

- complement components C3a and C5a
- reaction of IgE with antigen: IgE molecules are bound to the surface of mast cells via specific receptors, and when the IgE binds antigen the mast cells degranulate
- cytokines such as IL-1 and IL-8
- physical stimuli (heat, cold, trauma);
- neuropeptides produced by neuroendocrine cells, e.g. substance P
- some drugs, e.g. morphine.

When stimulated to degranulate, mast cells also metabolize arachidonic acid into inflammatory mediators such as prostaglandins. In these ways, mast cells are important effectors of the acute inflammatory response.

Macrophages

In acute inflammation, macrophages secrete cytokines, including IL-1 and TNF-α, and exhibit phagocytosis. However, they have a bigger role in chronic inflammation (Ch. 6).

6. Chronic inflammation

Questions
- What is chronic inflammation?
- How may chronic inflammation be manifest clinically?
- What are the major cells types involved in chronic inflammation and what are their roles?

Chronic inflammation is characterized by tissue damage and attempts at repair occurring simultaneously. It may follow acute inflammation, or it may occur ab initio without preceding acute inflammation. Examples of chronic inflammatory processes that develop without a preceding acute phase are:

- infection with organisms that are predominantly intracellular, e.g. tuberculosis, viruses
- presence of foreign body, e.g. suture materials, implanted prostheses, inhaled dusts
- many autoimmune diseases
- cellular rejection of transplants.

The inflammatory cells that characterize the chronic inflammatory response histologically are macrophages and their derivatives, lymphocytes, plasma cells and eosinophils. Pathologists refer to them as the 'chronic inflammatory cells'. Unless present in the tissue already, these cells are recruited to the site of inflammation by a process similar to that described for neutrophils in Ch. 5. Vascular events are involved in chronic inflammation, similar to those that occur in acute inflammation.

The role of macrophages
In addition to their phagocytic function, macrophages have important coordinating roles in chronic inflammation by virtue of their interactions with other inflammatory cells, antigen presentation and secretion of cytokines. They are an important component of the adaptive immune response and act to orchestrate many of its functions. Unlike neutrophils, macrophages are long lived and can persist for a long time. Macrophages in inflamed tissues are derived from blood monocytes produced in the bone marrow and are, therefore, part of the mononuclear phagocyte system (**reticuloendothelial system**). This system consists of the derivatives of monocytes and includes (Fig. 3.6.1):

- macrophages recruited to inflamed tissues from the bloodstream
- the fixed tissue macrophages such Kupffer cells in the liver, microglial cells in the brain and alveolar macrophages in the lungs
- specialized derivatives of macrophages such as epithelioid cells and multinucleate giant cells

- antigen-presenting dendritic cells, such as the Langerhans' cells of squamous epithelia and dendritic cells of lymph nodes
- osteoclasts.

Sometimes, two or more macrophages may attempt to ingest the same particle, in which case the cytoplasm of the cells fuses together to form large cells with many nuclei (**multinucleate giant cells**). This process typically occurs where the material is indigestible, for example:

- **Langhan giant cells:** bacteria such as mycobacteria can survive within macrophages; the giant cells that result often have a horse-shoe-like arrangement of nuclei (not the same as Langerhans' cells)
- **foreign body giant cells:** fragments of inert foreign material such as silica and surgical sutures are commonly surrounded by multinucleated giant cells; the nuclei are typically scattered randomly through the cytoplasm (Fig. 3.6.2)
- **Touton giant cells:** form in areas where large amounts of lipid break down; they are characterized by a central ring of nuclei and a peripheral zone of foamy cytoplasm containing lipid.

Epithelioid cells are macrophages that are specialized for secretory activities and have lost most of their phagocytic abilities. Their name is derived from a superficial resemblance to epithelial cells, which is imparted by their abundant eosinophilic cytoplasm. They often clump together to form granulomas. A **granuloma** is a collection of epithelioid macrophages together with variable numbers of other inflammatory cells (Fig. 3.6.3). Depending on the aetiology of the inflammatory process, granulomas may contain giant cells in addition to epithelioid cells. Examples of conditions

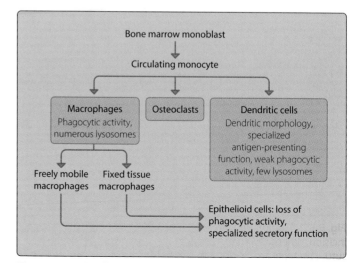

Fig. 3.6.1 Cells of the monocyte–macrophage system.

characterized by granulomatous inflammation are mycobacterial infections such as tuberculosis and leprosy, fungal infections, certain parasites, sarcoidosis, Crohn's disease, some drug reactions, and reactions to foreign material. Sometimes, the centre of the granuloma may become necrotic; a particular example of this phenomenon is the caseous necrosis seen in tuberculosis.

Sometimes, the term histiocyte is used for macrophages. It is a rather imprecise term and can be used for any macrophage except for the fixed tissue macrophages.

The role of lymphocytes

In inflamed tissues, **B-cells** are stimulated to differentiate into plasma cells and secrete immunoglobulins. **T-cells** have a variety of functions. In summary, the T-cells carrying the surface receptor CD4 (CD4 cells; helper T-cells) interact with antigen-presenting macrophages and secrete cytokines that influence the function of virtually all the other cells of the immune system. Helper T-cells can be divided broadly into two types: the first, Th1, secretes IL-1 and interferon-gamma and the second, Th2, secretes IL-4, IL-5 and IL-10. Their effects depend on this difference in cytokine production:

- **Th1 response**: macrophages are activated, plasma cells secrete IgG_2, and the Th2 response is inhibited
- **Th2 response**: eosinophils are activated, plasma cells secrete IgE, and the Th1 response is inhibited.

T-cells carrying the CD8 molecule (CD8 cells; suppressor/cytotoxic cells) also secrete cytokines, predominantly producing a Th1-type response. However, their principal function is to kill other cells (e.g. cells infected with virus).

The role of eosinophils

Eosinophils are recruited in parasitic infestations and in immune reactions mediated by IgE. The granules of eosinophils contain basic proteins that are toxic to parasites, such as major basic protein and eosinophil cationic protein.

Morphological appearances of chronic inflammation

Fibrosis is a common manifestation of the chronic inflammatory process. It may cause a visible scar or thickening of the wall of a hollow viscus, perhaps creating a stricture. Granulation tissue is also a marker of chronic inflammation. It can be seen in the bed of a chronic ulcer (an ulcer is defined as an abnormal breach of a mucosal surface). Necrosis may be present.

Microscopically, there will be varying numbers of any or all of the chronic inflammatory cells (i.e. macrophages, plasma cells, lymphocytes and eosinophils). Neutrophils may be present in small numbers, but if many neutrophils are visible the pathologist may use a term such as 'acute and chronic inflammation' or 'acute-on-chronic inflammation', depending on the clinical circumstances.

There are many different histological patterns of chronic inflammation. Although they are rarely entirely specific, they can provide clues to the aetiology of the inflammation. Therefore, given sufficient clinical information, the pathologist may be able to suggest likely causes of the inflammatory process observed in a specimen from a patient. For example, large numbers of eosinophils may suggest the presence of a parasite or an allergic reaction, while granulomas point to one of the causes of granulomatous inflammation.

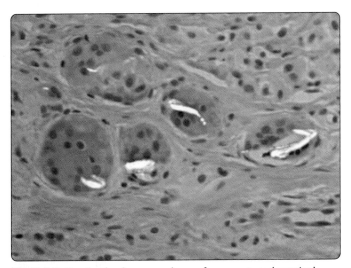

Fig. 3.6.2 Foreign body macrophages from a sutured surgical incision. When viewed under partially polarized light, fragments of suture material are visible within their cytoplasm. Macrophages like these are important in removing foreign material from the tissues.

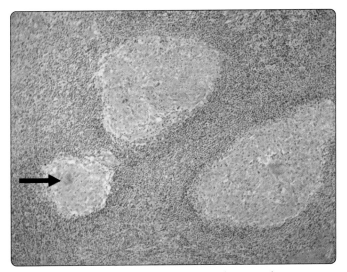

Fig. 3.6.3 Granulomas in the appendix. In this case, the granulomatous inflammation resulted from infection with *Yersinia pseudotuberculosis*. There are occasional multinucleated giant cells (arrow).

7. Organization, granulation tissue and fibrosis

Questions
- What is meant by the terms organization, granulation tissue and fibrosis?
- How do wounds heal?

Organization is the process by which granulation tissue replaces damaged tissue or inanimate material such as blood clot. The granulation tissue then matures into a scar. The term fibrosis is used for healing by scar formation via this mechanism. Organization occurs when:

- large amounts of fibrin or exudate cannot be removed by other means
- inflammation has caused tissue damage that cannot heal by resolution
- ischaemia has caused an infarct.

Components of granulation tissue

The three principal constituents of granulation tissue are endothelial cells, fibroblasts and myofibroblasts, and macrophages (Fig. 3.7.1). Other cells are also present in most cases, the type depending on the aetiology of the granulation tissue formation. For example, abundant inflammatory cells will be found in the granulation tissue at the base of a chronic peptic ulcer.

Endothelial cells grow into the exudate or dead tissue to vascularize it. This process of blood vessel formation is known as **angiogenesis** or neovascularization. The endothelial cells initially form solid cords, but they soon develop lumina and become capillaries. Indeed, the term granulation tissue comes from the granular appearance imparted by loops and coils of newly formed capillaries. The new endothelial cells are derived from two sources:

- sprouting from preexisting vessels adjacent to the injury
- endothelial precursor cells derived from the bone marrow; these cells are mobilized from the marrow and circulate to the site of injury, where they migrate into the tissues.

New arterioles and venules are formed as the proliferating capillaries become surrounded by pericytes and smooth muscle cells.

The **fibroblasts** and **myofibroblasts** produce matrix materials, in particular the collagen that will provide the strength of the scar. The myofibroblasts also have contractile abilities because their cytoplasm contains filaments similar to those in smooth muscle and they can draw the components of the developing scar together. As a result of myofibroblast contraction, the final scar may be much smaller than the original injury. (In H&E histological sections, myofibroblasts and fibroblasts look identical, but they can be distinguished by special techniques.)

Macrophages are required to dispose of dead tissue or unwanted material by phagocytosis. They also have an important role in coordinating the inflammatory response in the healing tissue.

Granulation tissue formation requires the migration, proliferation and differentiation of cells of many different types. Cytokines regulate these processes and control the activities of the cells. For example, vascular endothelial growth factor is secreted by many different cells and stimulates the sprouting of endothelial cells from preexisting vessels and also stimulates the release, proliferation and differentiation of endothelial precursor cells. Another function is to increase vascular permeability, promoting the exudation of plasma proteins in inflamed tissues.

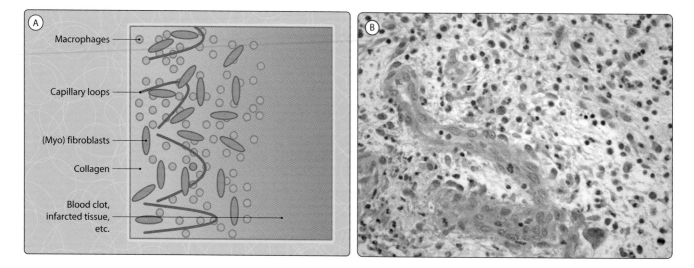

Fig. 3.7.1 Granulation tissue. (A) Components in granulation. (B) Oedematous connective tissue containing fibroblasts and inflammatory cells.

Healing by primary and secondary union

Two contrasting patterns of healing are termed primary and secondary union, also known as healing by first and second intention, respectively. The classical description of these patterns refers to healing in the skin and subcutaneous tissues, but similar principles apply elsewhere in the body.

Primary union occurs in a clean, incised wound with minimal tissue destruction if the edges of the wound are promptly drawn together and there is no significant bacterial contamination. A typical example is a wound made by a surgeon's scalpel and then sutured. Relatively little granulation tissue is produced under these circumstances, and scar formation is minimal.

Secondary union occurs in a wound that does not fulfil the criteria for healing by first intention: there is significant tissue destruction, the edges are not opposed, or there is infection or contamination with foreign material. In this case, granulation tissue forms in the base of the wound and grows to fill the defect. The result of this abundant granulation tissue formation is a large scar, contrasting with the minimal scarring of primary union.

Maturation of granulation tissue

With time, the granulation tissue becomes less cellular and the proportion of collagen increases. Eventually, the area is transformed into a scar of dense fibrous tissue (i.e. fibrosis). This mechanism of repair is versatile and efficient. However, the scar itself can cause disease.

Cosmetic problems. Cutaneous scars can be unsightly, especially if the scar tissue is excessive (a scar that stands proud of the skin surface is called a **hypertrophic scar**, and one that also extends beyond the site of original injury is called a **keloid**).

Adhesions. Organization of fibrinous exudates in serosal cavities may produce fibrous scars that stick the serosal surfaces together. These adhesions can produce complications, such as intestinal obstruction from peritoneal adhesions.

Luminal obstruction. Scarring in the wall of a hollow viscus can produce stricture (narrowing) that impedes the flow of intraluminal contents. Examples include gastric outflow obstruction from a peptic ulcer, and urethral stricture following infection of the urethra. In Fig. 3.7.2, fibrosis of the wall of the small intestine has caused a stricture.

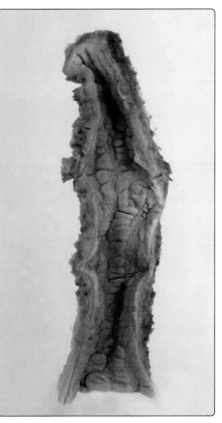

Fig. 3.7.2 Longitudinal section of a segment of small intestine with Crohn's disease. The wall of the intestine is diffusely thickened by fibrous scar tissue that has resulted from chronic inflammation and consequent tissue damage. The specimen also shows the cobblestone pattern of mucosal damage characteristic of Crohn's disease.

Limitation of movement. A scarred limb may have a restricted range of movement. Such an abnormality is called a **contracture**.

After the scar has formed, structural modifications of the collagen in the scar (e.g. increased cross-linking, increased fibre diameter) increase its tensile strength. This remodelling continues for months or years.

Note that granulation tissue is not to be confused with a granuloma. The latter is a collection of macrophages and, although granulation tissue can contain granulomas, the two terms are entirely distinct.

8. Chemical messengers important in inflammation

Questions
- How is the inflammatory response orchestrated?
- What are the main protein cascade systems involved in inflammation?

There are many chemicals important in inflammation. They are linked in a complex web of feedback mechanisms that control the inflammatory response. These chemicals can be divided into endogenous mediators that are produced by cells within the tissues and plasma proteins that circulate in the bloodstream.

Endogenous chemical mediators

The chemical mediators can either be released from granules where they are preformed and stored (e.g. histamine) or be synthesized on demand (e.g. the arachadonic acid derivatives prostaglandins, leukotrienes and lipoxins)

Histamine is mostly released from granules in mast cells, although eosinophils and platelets also contain some. Mast cells appear to be derived from circulating basophils, which are very similar cells. Histamine causes vascular dilatation and increased vascular permeability. It is quick acting and, therefore, it is important in acute inflammation.

Serotonin (5-hydroxytryptamine) is similar to histamine, but in humans it is found in platelets rather than mast cells.

Prostaglandins are a group of compounds having a range of effects; some increase vascular permeability, others induce platelet aggregation. The non-steroidal anti-inflammatory drugs (NSAIDs) inhibit enzymes involved in prostaglandin synthesis.

Leukotrienes are powerful chemotactic agents and cause vasoconstriction and leukocyte adhesion, and chemotaxis and activation of neutrophils and macrophages.

Lipoxins are arachadonic acid derivatives and have anti-inflammatory effects, tending to inhibit leukocyte activity.

Nitric oxide is a potent vasodilator and it also inhibits rolling and adhesion of leukocytes. It is synthesized by endothelial and inflammatory cells in response to cytokine stimulation.

Cytokines are a superfamily of inflammatory mediators produced at a site of injury and include interleukins (IL), interferons, colony-stimulating factors, growth factors, tumour necrosis factors (TNF) and chemokines.

Cytokines

The term cytokine is used for inflammatory mediators produced at a site of injury or inflammation that are not stored as preformed substances or prohormones but are produced when required via transcription and translation of the relevant genes.

They are polypeptides or glycoproteins of low molecular weight and act by binding to receptors of target cells, generally affecting gene transcription via second messengers. Cytokines can be divided into a number of groups depending on their principal functions, but many have multiple roles and could be included in several different groups. Some, like TNF-α activate phagocytes, while others, like IL-2 and transforming growth factor (TGF) beta regulate lymphocyte growth, differentiation and activity. The chemokines are cytokines with chemoattractant properties and are responsible for the migration of inflammatory cells by chemotaxis; they can also activate leukocytes. Cytokines can have autocrine, paracrine or endocrine effects; an example of the last is the fever that accompanies inflammation.

A useful way of thinking about cytokines is to divide them into **pro-inflammatory cytokines** (e.g. TNF-α, IL-1, IL-2, IL-6) that upregulate inflammatory responses, and **anti-inflammatory cytokines** (e.g. IL-4, IL-10 and TGF-β) that act as a brake on inflammation and actively terminate the process. However, because of the complex nature of inflammation control, some cytokines can be pro-inflammatory in some circumstances and anti-inflammatory in others. Therapeutic manipulation of cytokines has the potential to help patients with a wide variety of inflammatory diseases, and research in this area has resulted in drugs such as infliximab, an antibody directed against TNF-α. Infliximab and related drugs inhibit TNF-α and can be used to treat conditions such as Crohn's disease and rheumatoid arthritis.

Plasma proteins

There are four cascade systems in the plasma that are involved in inflammatory processes. In each system, the inactive precursors are converted into active mediators in a stepwise fashion. There are a number of features inherent in such cascade systems:

- the precursors circulate in inactive form, ready for immediate conversion to the active form when required
- the conversion reactions are subject to feedback control
- each step results in an amplification of the response, since one enzyme molecule can activate many substrate molecules
- a variety of end-products can be produced from a single initial activation.

The four systems are interrelated and are shown in Fig. 3.8.1.

Coagulation system. This results in the formation of **fibrin**, a major component of the inflammatory exudate. It can be initiated when factor XII is activated by contact with extracellular matrix (intrinsic activation) or by the activation of factor VII by lipoproteins released from damaged cells (extrinsic activation). In addition, **thrombin**, the enzyme that produces fibrin from circulating fibrinogen, forms a link between the inflammatory response and the coagulation cascade. It does this by binding to protease-activated receptors on platelets, endothelial cells and other cells. The binding to these receptors promotes many aspects of the inflammatory response, including the production of cytokines, nitric oxide and prostaglandins, and upregulation of endothelial adhesion molecules.

Fibrinolytic system. This cascade acts as a counterbalance to the coagulation cascade. It is initiated by activated factor XII and by plasminogen activators released by endothelial cells and leukocytes. Plasminogen is the inactive precursor of **plasmin**, which, in turn, lyses insoluble fibrin into soluble fibrin degradation products, also known as fibrin split products, thus allowing the clot to dissolve. However, plasmin also has other functions. In particular, it cleaves factor C3 in the complement cascade.

Complement system. The principal functions of the complement proteins are in defence against microorganisms. The cascade is activated by a number of mechanisms, including antibody–antigen complexes (**classical pathway**) and substances produced by microbes, e.g. endotoxin (**alternative pathway**). Whatever the activating mechanism, C3 is cleaved into two fragments: C3b, which remains where it was formed by binding covalently, and C3a, which diffuses away.

Further activation steps follow the production of C3b, with the ultimate production of the **membrane attack complex**, which breaches the cell membrane. The functions of the complement system are first to produce the membrane attack complex and, second, to produce active fragments of complement components. These fragments have a number of functions in the inflammatory response. For example, C5a is a potent chemoattractant for leukocytes while both C3a and C5a stimulate histamine release from mast cells.

Kinin system. The kinins (e.g. **bradykinin**) are produced from inactive precursors called kininogens by the enzyme kallikrein. They generally cause dilation of vessels, increased vascular permeability and pain. The cascade is initiated by activated factor XII, which converts prekallikrien into the active proteolytic form kallikrein. The plasma glycoprotein high-molecular-weight kininogen is a substrate for kallikrein, which cleaves it to produce bradykinin. In addition, kallikrien activates factor XII. This ability means that a positive feedback loop is established, whereby kallikrein that has been activated by factor XII itself activates more factor XII. The resulting autocatalytic pathway is a powerful means of amplifying the initial stimulus. Bradykinin itself stimulates plasmin activation; it also promotes synthesis of prostacyclin (prostaglandin I_2) and nitric oxide, and inhibits platelet function.

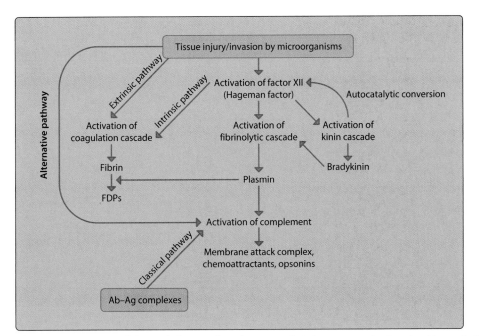

Fig. 3.8.1 Summary of the main interactions between the plasma proteins involved in acute inflammation. Note that activated factor XII directly or indirectly initiates all four of these plasma protein cascades. Ab–Ag, antibody–antigen; FDP, fibrin degradation products.

9. Causes of cell injury

Questions
- How may cells and tissues become injured?
- Why is cellular injury important in the development of disease?

There is a wide variety of agents that can cause cell damage. Whatever the cause, if the injury is relatively minor the cell may be able to repair itself and return to normal. This is **reversible injury**; it may be characterized morphologically at the light microscopic level by cellular swelling (called hydropic change or vacuolar degeneration) or by fatty change, and at the ultrastructural level by blebbing of the cell membrane, abnormalities of mitochondria and endoplasmic reticulum, and disaggregation of nuclear structures. However, if the initial insult to the cell is severe or prolonged, an **irreversible injury** will occur and the cell will die by apoptosis or necrosis. The factors that determine which pathway is followed are complex and not entirely understood but it seems that damage to cell membranes promotes death by necrosis rather than apoptosis. These pathways are illustrated in Fig. 3.9.1 (see also Ch. 10).

The causes of cell injury can be classified into hypoxia (lack of oxygen), physical agents, chemical agents, microorganisms and immune reactions.

Hypoxia

In clinical practice, cell damage caused by reduced oxygen supply is usually a consequence of reduced blood flow (**ischaemia**). A zone of necrosis caused by ischaemia is an **infarct**. The pathways involved in hypoxic cell damage are summarized in Fig. 3.9.2. The initiating factor is reduced availability of energy in the form of ATP, which causes the ion pumps to fail and the metabolic processes of the cell to increase production of reactive oxygen species. The latter directly damage cell components such as membranes, while the failure of ion pumps causes activation of proteases and phospholipases as the concentration of calcium within the cell rises. As the integrity of membranes breaks down, more calcium is released from the endoplasmic reticulum, and digestive enzymes are released from lysosomes. Cell death occurs by necrosis or apoptosis, depending on the severity of the injury. Cerebral neurons die after only a few minutes if the blood supply is cut off; other cells survive longer (e.g. liver cells can last an hour or two).

In principle, reduced blood flow through a vessel can occur through anatomical obstruction of flow or through changes in the way blood flows through the vessel. These mechanisms can be classified as follows. Note the correct use of terminology: occlusion means complete obstruction and stenosis means narrowing.

Intraluminal obstruction. The principal intraluminal lesions are **thrombi** and **emboli** (Ch. 37). Occasionally, other diseases can cause intraluminal obstruction. For example, in **cryoglobulinaemia** capillaries can be blocked by precipitation of abnormal proteins at low temperatures, and in **sickle cell anaemia** small vessels can be plugged by aggregations of erythrocytes.

Lesions of the vessel wall. By far the most common disease causing significant ischaemia in industrialized nations is **atherosclerosis**. It only affects arteries and is often complicated by superimposed thrombosis. **Vasculitis** causes narrowing of vessels and can also be complicated by superimposed thrombosis. Vasculitis and atherosclerosis are covered in Chs 15 and 34, respectively. Sometimes, **spasm** of vessels occurs as a result of contraction of the smooth muscle of the media. Reduction in nitric oxide production by the endothelium as a result of injury is an important mechanism of arterial spasm. The resulting stenosis can cause symptoms (e.g. Prinzmetal angina).

Lesions outside the wall. Compression of a vessel from the outside can cause obstruction to flow. Veins, being thin walled, are more prone to outside compression than arteries. Compression could occur as a result of a growing cyst or tumour pressing on the vessel or through squeezing of

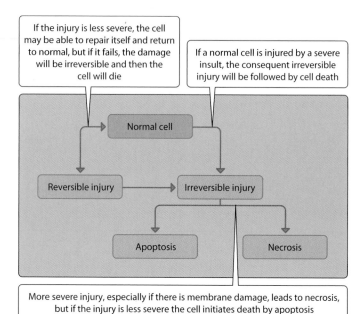

Fig. 3.9.1 Pathways of cell death.

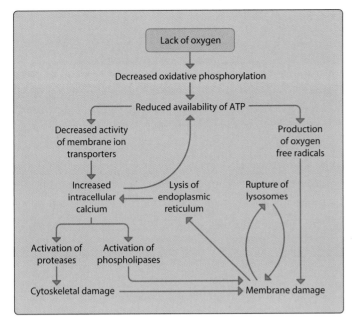

Fig. 3.9.2 Pathogenesis of hypoxic cell injury.

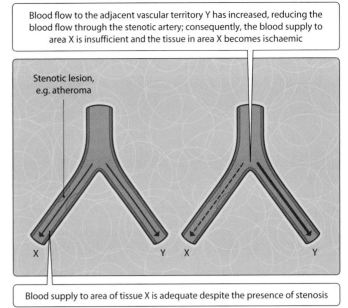

Fig. 3.9.3 Vascular steal.

the vasculature in torsion, herniation, volvulus or intussusception.

Abnormalities of blood flow. **Hyperviscosity** of the blood occurs in some conditions, for example in polycythaemia and hypergammaglobulinaemia. It predisposes to thrombosis and impairs flow through stenotic vessels. **Vascular steal** occurs when a stenotic artery allows sufficient flow at rest, but when blood flow increases to neighbouring territories as a result of increased demand, the flow of blood through the narrowed vessel becomes inadequate (Fig. 3.9.3). The other arteries are said to 'steal' the blood from the narrowed artery as blood is diverted through them.

Physical agents

Physical phenomena damaging cells include:

- **heat**: denaturation of proteins
- **cold**: vasoconstriction associated with severe cold can produce hypoxia; if tissue freezes, ice crystals disrupt the cells causing frostbite
- **trauma**: disrupts cells
- **electricity**: disrupts cells and may also cause heat damage
- **ionizing radiation**: electromagnetic radiation and energetic particles that strip electrons from atoms and molecules can damage cell components, for example sunburn from ultraviolet light; additionally, damage to DNA by ionizing radiation can cause neoplasia.

Chemical agents

Chemical agents include inorganic chemicals such as cyanide and organic chemicals such as toxins and drugs. The effects can be highly specific, for example cyanide inhibiting cytochrome oxidase, or they can be more generalized, for example phospholipid damage in chronic alcoholism. Chemicals may cause widespread disruption of membranes, and protein damage can affect both the cytoskeleton and enzymes. Free radicals produced by various metabolic processes are highly reactive and can cause damage to cells. Toxins produced by venomous animals can directly damage cells or can also have an effect through ischaemia by causing severe vasoconstriction.

Microorganisms

The inflammatory reaction to infection causes damage to adjacent host tissues through an 'innocent bystander' effect. In addition, bacteria produce toxins that damage cells directly. Viruses have a cytopathic effect on infected cells; the replication cycle of the the virus damages the infected cell and ultimately kills it.

Immune reactions

Immune reactions can occur in the presence of microorganisms, as part of autoimmune diseases or in transplant rejection. Cell damage occurs through activation of inflammatory processes or as a direct result of activation of cytotoxic T-cells or natural killer cells.

10. Cell death

Questions
- What are the mechanisms involved in cell death?
- How may cellular death be manifest clinically?

Cell death can be divided into three main types: apoptosis, necrosis and autolysis. Chapter 9 discussed the causes of cell death.

Apoptosis

Apoptosis, or programmed cell death, is internally regulated by the cell and is characterized morphologically by the production of membrane-bound apoptotic bodies (Fig. 3.10.1). It can occur as a normal phenomenon, as discussed in Ch. 2. In pathological circumstances, apoptosis can be involved in many different ways: for example loss of CD4 T-cells in infection by the human deficiency virus (HIV), reduction in cell number in pathological atrophy, and cell loss by apoptosis rather than necrosis at the edge of infarcts. In neoplasia, there is *insufficient* apoptosis: the balance between apoptosis and cell proliferation is disturbed so that cell proliferation exceeds cell loss and the net result is tumour growth.

Mechanism of apoptosis

Apoptosis can be divided into three stages: initiation, execution and phagocytosis.

1. **Initiation.** Examples of initiating stimuli include intrinsic activation of genes, as seen during embryogenesis, changes in cell–cell or cell–matrix interactions, changes in stimulation by soluble mediators such as growth factors and hormones, injurious agents (hypoxia, toxins etc.), and release of granzymes from cytotoxic T-cells. These triggers initiate cell signalling mechanisms that ultimately result in procaspase 8 or procaspase 9 being transformed into their active form. The initiating systems are interlinked and rather complex, but in essence there are two main pathways. First is the **extrinsic (death receptor) pathway**. Important in immune reactions, this pathway is triggered by the binding of ligands to death receptors such as Fas expressed on the surface of the cell. The initial caspase to be activated is caspase 8. Second is the **intrinsic (mitochondrial) pathway**. The key stage is an increase in permeability of the mitochondrial membrane, releasing cytochrome *c* into the cytoplasm. Mitochondrial permeability is controlled by the Bcl-2 family of proteins. The initiator caspase in this pathway is caspase 9.

2. **Execution**. The caspase cascade, initiated by caspase 8 or 9, is the final common pathway that leads to the production of apoptotic bodies. Caspases are normally present as inactive proenzymes, but when the initiator caspases are activated the cascade is triggered, culminating in the activation of executioner caspases that act on cellular components to bring about cell death. For example, they cleave components of the cytoskeleton, causing the cell to shrink and ultimately break up into apoptotic bodies. They also activate a DNase that cleaves DNA at internucleosomal sites, breaking it up into fragments 180–200 base-pairs in length. During the production of apoptotic bodies, the plasma membrane is preserved so that cytoplasmic contents do not leak out. The important steps on these pathways are regulated by inhibitors and enhancers that modulate the processes involved.

3. **Phagocytosis.** The apoptotic bodies are disposed of by phagocytosis (Fig. 3.10.1D). Although macrophages are important in performing this task, other cells that do not normally have phagocytic abilities (e.g. adjacent epithelial cells) are able to do so as well. This process is promoted by the expression of molecules on the surface of the apoptotic bodies that act as ligands for other cells, allowing them to bind to the apoptotic bodies and ingest them. Neighbouring cells may migrate or proliferate to fill the space that was occupied by the deleted cell.

Necrosis

Necrosis is the passive death of cells in the living organism through irreversible cell injury. The process is not regulated by the cell. Unlike apoptosis, which can occur in normal tissues, necrosis only occurs in pathological circumstances. It is characterized by damage to cell membranes that allows cytoplasmic contents to escape; the release of cytoplasmic components into the bloodstream can be a useful clinical indicator of necrosis. For example, circulating levels of myocardial enzymes and troponins are used as blood tests for myocardial infarction. Unlike apoptosis, necrosis stimulates an inflammatory reaction and affects sheets of cells rather than individual, scattered cells. The main differences between apoptosis and necrosis are summarized in Table 3.10.1. Since the causes of apoptosis and necrosis overlap, they often occur together in damaged tissues. Morphologically, necrosis can be divided into four main types:

Coagulative necrosis. This is the commonest type and is characterized by persistence of the basic outline of the cells; as a result, the architecture of the necrotic tissue can be discerned histologically for some time.

Colliquative (liquefactive) necrosis. Necrosis in the brain and spinal cord is characterized by rapid loss of cell outlines associated with liquefaction of the tissue (Fig. 3.57.3).

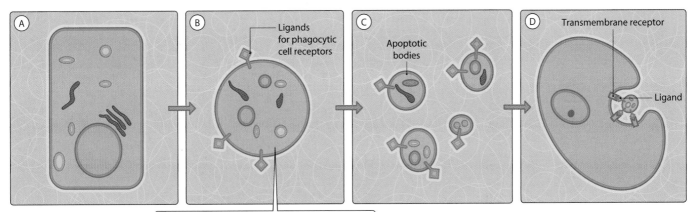

Fig. 3.10.1 Morphology of apoptosis. (A) A normal cell begins to round up; (B) increased cytoplasmic eosinophilia and breakdown of cell components; (C) the cell itself disintegrates into membrane-bound apoptotic bodies; (D) phagocytosis of the apoptotic bodies.

Table 3.10.1 APOPTOSIS AND NECROSIS CONTRASTED

Apoptosis	Necrosis
Physiological or pathological	Always pathological
Membrane integrity preserved	Membranes breached with loss of cytoplasm into the extracellular fluid
No inflammation	Inflammatory response
Affects single cells	Affects contiguous cells
Active process: requires protein synthesis and consumes ATP	Passive process

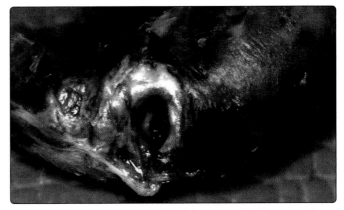

Fig. 3.10.2 Gangrenous necrosis of the appendix. The organ has ruptured through the weakened wall.

Caseous necrosis. The prototype of caseous necrosis is seen in tuberculosis. Indeed, when a pathologist uses the term caseous, the usual implication is that mycobacterial infection is the cause. Caseation can occur occasionally in other circumstances (e.g. histoplasmosis). To the naked eye, caseation is soft, pale grey or white material resembling cream cheese (hence the name). Histologically, there is rapid loss of cell outlines producing granular debris (Fig. 3.43.1).

Gangrenous necrosis. The term gangrene does not have a precise use in medical practice, but it usually implies infection of necrotic tissue. It is characterized by green, blue or black discolouration, and a foul smell resulting from the metabolic activity of bacteria (Fig. 3.10.2). There are three types of gangrene: dry (gradual reduction in blood supply; Ch. 34), gas (abundant from gas-producing bacteria) and wet (dead cells lyse releasing fluid that is infected by bacteria). Sometimes, a highly pathogenic organism such as *Clostridium*

perfringens can cause gangrene by invading viable tissue but more commonly, tissue that is already dead is colonized by saprophytic organisms that then start to digest it.

Autolysis

When a pathologist uses the term autolysis it is generally to describe passive cell death occurring elsewhere than in the living organism. That is, it refers to cell death occurring either postmortem or in tissue that has been surgically removed. Autolysis resembles necrosis in many respects, but there is no inflammatory response because it does not occur in the context of a living organism. The release of digestive enzymes from lysosomes in the dead cells is an important mechanism in autolysis. If a surgical specimen or biopsy is not adequately fixed with formalin or other fixative solution, autolytic changes in the tissues alter and disguise the morphological appearances, and may prevent the pathologist from giving a meaningful diagnosis.

11. Tissue degenerations

Questions
- What substances accumulate in tissue degeneration?
- How do these changes reflect pathogenesis?
- How can recognizing them be useful to the pathologist?

There are a number of miscellaneous pathological changes characterized by the abnormal accumulation of various substances in tissues. Sometimes called **tissue degenerations**, they can provide important information about the underlying disease process.

Calcification

Pathological calcification is abnormal deposition of calcium salts plus small quantities of other minerals. Macroscopically, calcification is white or pale grey, and it produces a hard or gritty feeling to palpation. Calcium is opaque to X-rays and can be seen radiologically. Histologically, calcium is basophilic with haematoxylin stain (Fig. 3.11.1); it also takes up other dyes. Heavily calcified tissues cannot be processed in the laboratory using routine paraffin wax methods so the tissue must be embedded in a hard medium such as acrylic or epoxy resin, or decalcified so it becomes soft. In long-standing calcification, osseous metaplasia can produce heterotopic bone within the calcified tissue.

Pathological calcification can be described as dystrophic or metastatic. **Dystrophic calcification** occurs in abnormal tissues in the presence of normal serum calcium. Most commonly, it is

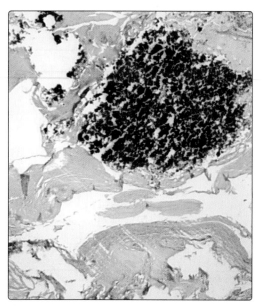

Fig. 3.11.1 Mucin with dystrophic calcification. The calcium is the dark blue material in the upper part of the figure. The mucin was produced by a mucinous carcinoma of the appendix and is the pale blue material surrounding the calcification. H&E stain.

encountered in necrotic tissue, for example caseous necrosis, the necrotic cores of atheromatous plaques, and areas of necrosis in cancers and old infarcts. Other places in which calcification may be found are old thrombi and abnormal heart valves. **Metastatic calcification** occurs in normal tissues as a result of hypercalcaemia. The calcium salts can be deposited in many different tissues, especially in the walls of arteries. If the kidneys are affected (nephrocalcinosis), renal failure can occur.

The chemical reactions causing the precipitation of calcium salts in the tissues are not well understood, but recent evidence suggests nanobacteria may have a role. Nanobacteria are extremely small Gram-negative bacteria that accumulate calcium phosphate on their surfaces. They have been associated with biomineralization in several different circumstances, including kidney stones and tumour calcification.

Amyloid

Amyloid is abnormal protein with a β-pleated sheet structure that is deposited in the extracellular space. The protein is derived from a normal precursor protein, but abnormal proteolysis gives rise to the β-pleated sheet form. Macroscopically, amyloid in large amounts gives organs a firm, waxy appearance. Microscopically, it has a homogenous eosinophilic appearance on H&E stains. Histochemical reactions are useful in diagnosis; for example, amyloid is positive with Congo red and exhibits an apple-green colour when the Congo red section is observed through crossed polarizing filters (Fig. 3.11.2A). Under the electron microscope, amyloid presents a characteristic fibrillar appearance.

Most amyloid deposits also contain glycoproteins, such as P component. Typically, approximately 95% of the material is amyloid protein and 5% P-component and other glycoproteins.

Amyloidosis can be described as systemic, affecting many different tissues, or localized, confined to one tissue (Table 3.11.1). The most important clinical sequelae from systemic amyloidosis usually result from renal involvement, producing nephrotic syndrome or chronic renal failure, or cardiac involvement, producing arrhythmias or a restrictive cardiomyopathy.

Hyaline change

Hyaline change is not a specific term and is used descriptively by pathologists for a variety of homogenous eosinophilic materials with a glassy, refractile look. It comes from the Greek word for glass, *hyalos*. For example, Mallory bodies in the liver have a hyaline appearance and deposits of proteins in renal tubules are called hyaline casts. The walls of arterioles in long-standing diabetes and hypertension become hyalinized.

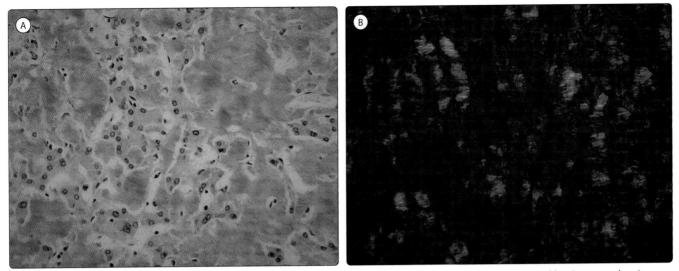

Fig. 3.11.2 Amyloidosis of the liver. (A) Massive accumulations of amyloid in liver sinusoids are demonstrated by Congo red stain. (B) Under polarized light, the stained amyloid exhibits apple-green birefringence.

Table 3.11.1 AMYLOID PROTEINS

Underlying condition	Precursor protein	Type of amyloid	Disease produced by the amyloid
Systemic amyloidosis			
Myeloma (or other monoclonal B-cell proliferation)	Immunoglobulin light chains	AL	Primary amyloidosis (localized production can cause an amyloid tumour)
Chronic inflammatory conditions (e.g. rheumatoid arthritis, tuberculosis, bronchiectasis)	SAA	AA	Secondary amyloidosis
Chronic haemodialysis for renal failure	β_2-Microglobulin	Aβ_2m	Haemodialysis-associated amyloidosis
Several rare hereditary forms of amyloidosis	SAA or TTR	AA or ATTR	Several types, e.g. familial Mediterranean fever (AA) and familial amyloid polyneuropathy (ATTR)
Localized amyloidosis			
Abnormal cleavage of APP	APP	β-Amyloid protein	Alzheimer's disease
Ageing, or inherited abnormality of TTR	TTR	ATTR	Senile cardiac amyloid
Endocrine neoplasia	Hormone (e.g. calcitonin in medullary carcinoma of thyroid)	Abnormal hormone	Amyloid deposits in endocrine neoplasms

SAA, serum amyloid-associated protein; APP, amyloid precursor protein; TTR, transthyretin.

Glycogen

Glycogen can be recognized histologically using the periodic acid–Schiff (PAS) reaction. It can accumulate in the cells of certain tumours, and occasionally identifying glycogen in a tumour may help with diagnosis. The glycogen storage diseases, or glycogenoses, are rare genetic disorders where glycogen accumulates in massive amounts within tissues causing secondary cell injury.

Myxomatous change

Mucins, like glycogen, stain positively with the PAS method. A diastase–PAS stain will distinguish mucin from glycogen as only glycogen is digested by diastase. Mucins are secretory products of many glandular epithelia and important components of the intercellular matrix, where they are produced by fibroblasts, chondroblasts and osteoblasts. An increase in the mucoid (myxoid) ground substance of connective tissue is called mucoid, or myxomatous, change. It is a non-specific degenerative phenomenon that can be a feature of a number of diseases, including Marfan syndrome, hypothyroidism, floppy mitral valve and ganglion cysts. Some neoplasms are characterized by a myxoid ground substance (e.g. myxofibrosarcoma and cardiac myxoma). Mucin also accumulates in the tissues in the rare genetic defects of mucopolysaccharide metabolism called the mucopolysaccharidoses.

12. Abnormal pigment deposition

Questions
- What pigments can be deposited under pathological circumstances?
- How does the presence of these pigments reflect the pathogenesis of the disease?
- How can finding these pigments be useful diagnostically?

Haemosiderin

Haemosiderin is a golden-brown pigment derived from the breakdown of haemoglobin. It can be demonstrated in tissue sections by the Prussian blue reaction, which is utilized in histological stains such as Perls stain. Small amounts are normal in the bone marrow, but otherwise its presence is usually pathological.

Localized haemosiderin deposition occurs in inflamed tissues from the breakdown of haemoglobin in extravasated red blood cells. The haemosiderin is taken up by macrophages (Fig. 3.12.1). The presence of this pigment is used by pathologists as an indicator that inflammation has occurred, and it may be mentioned in histopathology reports for this reason.

If there is systemic iron overload, haemosiderin is deposited in many organs and tissues. Causes include haemolytic anaemia, recurrent blood transfusions, increased absorption of iron from the intestine, and inherited disorders of iron metabolism. The most common inherited disorder of iron metabolism is a homozygous recessive disorder called **hereditary haemochromatosis** and caused by a mutation of the gene *HFE*. The consequence is failure of the normal regulation of iron absorption from the intestine so that excessive quantities of iron are absorbed from the gut lumen. Large amounts of iron in the liver, heart, pancreas and skin can cause hepatic fibrosis, heart failure, diabetes and skin pigmentation, respectively.

Pathologists tend to use the term **haemosiderosis** for the presence of iron in the tissues, while the disease caused by the iron is called **haemochromatosis**.

Lipofuscin

Lipofuscin is an intracellular brown-yellow pigment that accumulates in many different cells with age. It is sometimes called the wear-and-tear pigment based on the assumption that it represents the accumulation with time of cell constituents that are indigestible to lysosomes. The result is a brown residue within the cell that increases as the cell ages. The liver and heart often contain deposits. Its presence is not believed to be harmful. The term ceroid is used for a brown pigment that is probably just a variety of lipofuscin.

Melanin

Melanin is a normal pigment in the skin, hair, uveal tract, substantia nigra and elsewhere, and melanin and melanin-like pigments can also be deposited in pathological circumstances. In Addison's disease, there is a generalized increase in melanin in the skin, particularly in light-exposed areas. Malignant melanoma is a neoplasm of melanin-producing cells; it is a common skin cancer and most lesions are characterized by melanin production (Fig. 3.12.2). Occasionally, malignant melanomas do not produce

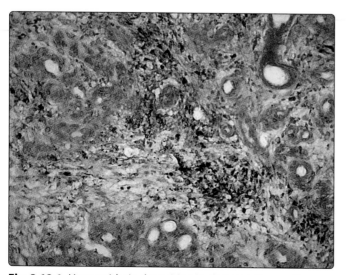

Fig. 3.12.1 Haemosiderin deposition in chronic inflammation. The Perls stain turns the haemosiderin blue.

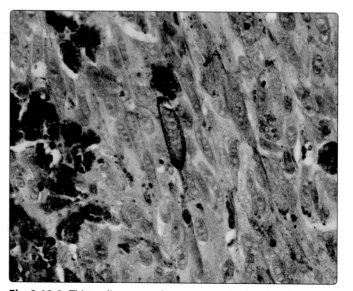

Fig. 3.12.2 This malignant melanoma contains large amounts of brown melanin pigment.

melanin; they are called amelanotic malignant melanomas. **Melanosis coli** is characterized by the deposition of melanin-like pigment in the mucosa of the colon, imparting a brown appearance. It appears to be harmless and is often associated with the use of purgatives.

Bilirubin

Bilirubin is a bile pigment that accumulates in jaundice. Unconjugated bilirubin is poorly soluble in water and most of it in the circulation is bound to albumin. Conjugated bilirubin is produced by combining bilirubin with glucuronides; the process occurs in the liver and renders the bilirubin readily soluble in water so it can be excreted in the bile. Unconjugated bilirubin accumulates when there is excess production of bilirubin or when there is a failure of hepatic conjugation. Conjugated bilirubin accumulates when there is a failure of secretion by hepatocytes or an obstruction to bile flow. Because conjugated bilirubin is soluble in water, the excess can be excreted in the urine. Therefore, dark urine is a symptom of conjugated hyperbilirubinaemia.

The principal causes of jaundice are summarized in Table 3.12.1. It shows the causes divided into prehepatic, hepatic and posthepatic types depending on the main site of the lesion: before the bilirubin enters the hepatocytes, in the hepatocytes themselves, or after the bile has been secreted into the biliary tree, respectively. Prehepatic jaundice is predominantly unconjugated while posthepatic jaundice is predominantly conjugated bilirubin. Hepatic jaundice can show either conjugated or unconjugated hyperbilirubinaemia; sometimes there is a mixed picture representing a failure of both conjugation and excretion by the damaged hepatocytes. In clinical practice, the most common causes of jaundice are haemolytic anaemia, hepatitis and extrahepatic biliary outflow obstruction.

Exogenous pigments

Pigments originating outside the body are called exogenous to distinguish them from pigments produced by the cells themselves. The two main routes by which exogenous pigments enter the body are via inhalation and through the skin. The commonest inhaled pigment is carbon from air pollution or coal dust. This material accumulates in the lungs producing a blackening called **anthracosis**, but if the accumulations are severe and associated with inflammation, the disease that results is coalworker's pneumoconiosis (Ch. 46). The way in which pigments are introduced via the skin is by tattooing. In a tattoo, the fine pigment particles are taken up by macrophages in the dermis and subcutis, where they remain indefinitely.

Table 3.12.1 COMMON CAUSES OF JAUNDICE

Type of jaundice	Pathogenesis	Predominant type of hyperbilirubinaemia	Examples
Prehepatic	Excess bilirubin production	Unconjugated	Haemolytic anaemia; reabsorption of blood from gastrointestinal haemorrhage
Hepatic	Defective hepatocyte function	Unconjugated	Neonatal jaundice; Gilbert syndrome; drugs affecting bile pigment uptake or conjugation
		Conjugated	Drugs affecting bile pigment excretion; cirrhosis; hepatitis (viral, autoimmune, alcoholic, etc.)
Posthepatic (cholestatic)	Damage to intrahepatic bile ducts	Conjugated	Certain drugs; primary biliary cirrhosis; primary sclerosing cholangitis; graft-versus-host disease
	Extrahepatic biliary obstruction	Conjugated	Gallstones; carcinoma of head of pancreas, extrahepatic biliary tree or ampulla of Vater; liver flukes; extrahepatic biliary atresia; strictures from previous surgery

13. Shock

Questions
- What is meant in medical terms by the word 'shock'?
- What are the causes of shock?
- How may shock be life threatening?

Shock can mean anything from a frightening or unexpected event to a fatal collapse of the body's circulation. Physiological shock is a dramatic reduction in blood flow that, if left untreated, can lead to collapse, coma and even death. Our favourite definition is 'systemic hypoperfusion owing to a reduction in either cardiac output or the effective circulating blood volume'. It is associated with hypotension. The clinical features of shock are caused by the cellular hypoxia resulting from reduced tissue perfusion. If relatively mild, the hypoxia causes reversible tissue injury. If severe or prolonged, irreversible cell damage occurs.

Pathogenesis

Shock can be classified according to pathogenesis into a number of types (Table 3.13.1). Hypovolaemic, cardiogenic and septic shock are the most common types.

Hypovolaemic shock

The responses of the body to hypovolaemia can be understood as evolutionary adaptations to preserve life in the face of severe haemorrhage from traumatic injuries. When blood is lost, for example through severing of a major artery, the baroreceptor reflexes are stimulated, catecholamines are secreted, the renin–angiotensin–aldosterone system is activated, and antidiuretic hormone is released. The consequences are:
- an increase in heart rate and cardiac output
- generalized peripheral vasoconstriction to maintain blood pressure despite the diminished blood volume
- diversion of blood from less vital organs to the brain and heart (which occurs because the vessels of the brain and heart are less sensitive to sympathetic vasoconstriction and, therefore, maintain their calibre)
- renal retention of salt and water to increase plasma volume.

Unless the shock is corrected, anaerobic respiration in underperfused tissues causes accumulation of lactic acid. This metabolic lactic acidosis adversely affects the vasoconstrictor response of vessels and blood begins to pool in the peripheral circulation. Blood pressure and cardiac output diminish further, and hypoxic damage worsens. Organ failure becomes apparent.

Cardiogenic shock

Cardiogenic shock occurs when the heart is severely damaged—by a major heart attack, for example—and is no longer able to pump blood around the body properly (acute pump failure), causing very low blood pressure. The term is usually taken to include extrinsic compression of the myocardium caused by tamponade and outflow obstruction owing to pulmonary embolism. The responses of the body are similar to those observed in hypovolaemic shock.

Septic shock

The pathogenesis of septic shock is complicated. It occurs when an overwhelming bacterial infection causes blood pressure to drop. Typically, it results from serious infection with Gram-negative bacteria such as *Escherichia coli, Klebsiella* or *Pseudomonas* spp. Toxic shock syndrome is a rare but severe illness caused by certain strains of *Staphylococcus aureus*. The bacteria release bacterial wall lipopolysaccharides, also known as **endotoxins**, which cause inflammation by activating macrophages and neutrophils and initiating the alternative complement pathway and the extrinsic coagulation pathway. Sometimes, similar lipopolysaccharides molecules are released from Gram-positive bacteria and fungi. If large amounts of lipopolysaccharides are present, there will be massive activation of inflammatory cells with release of large quantities of cytokines into the circulation. Although these cytokines at low levels have beneficial effects by playing their part in host defence (Ch. 8), at high levels they cause:
- systemic vasodilatation such that the circulating blood volume cannot fill the greatly increased volume of the vascular bed, resulting in hypotension
- reduced myocardial contractility and cardiac output
- increased capillary permeability, resulting in loss of intravascular volume to the extravascular space
- maldistribution of flow owing to microvascular abnormalities: blood flow does not reflect metabolic need
- disseminated intravascular coagulation (DIC).

The hypotension, reduced cardiac output and increased capillary permeability are responsible for septic shock, while the maldistribution of flow further compromises tissue perfusion. The DIC can complicate the clinical picture.

Two phases of septic shock are recognized. In the initial **hyperdynamic phase**, there is reduction in systemic vascular resistance but the cardiac output is maintained. Indeed, the cardiac output may rise somewhat in response to tachycardia and plasma volume expansion by retention of salt and water. Nevertheless, the cardiac output is insufficient to perfuse the dilated systemic circulation adequately. As sepsis worsens, the condition

Table 3.13.1 COMPARISON OF THE DIFFERENT TYPES OF SHOCK

Type of shock	Cardiac output	Behaviour of systemic vessels	Examples
Hypovolaemic	Reduced	Secondary vasoconstriction	Haemorrhage from a severed major artery; loss of plasma in extensive burns; loss of fluid from the colon in cholera
Cardiogenic	Reduced	Secondary vasoconstriction	Myocardial infarction; rupture of a cardiac valve cusp; arrhythmia; cardiac tamponade; pulmonary embolism
Septic	Reduced (after initial rise)	Dilatation (constriction later)	Microbial infection
Anaphylactic	Secondary increase	Widespread dilatation	Allergy
Neurogenic	Secondary increase	Widespread dilatation	Spinal cord injury

enters the **hypodynamic phase**. Vasoconstriction occurs and the cardiac output declines. A marked lactic acidosis is typical.

Anaphylactic shock

Anaphylactic shock results from an acute systemic type 1 hypersensitivity reaction in individuals sensitized to an antigen; common triggers include bee and wasp stings, nuts, shellfish, eggs, latex and certain medications, including penicillin. There is systemic vascular dilatation causing hypotension and inadequate tissue perfusion. Cardiac function is normal. In addition to hypotension, the anaphylactic reaction may include bronchospasm, urticaria and laryngeal oedema.

Neurogenic shock

If the spinal cord is damaged, there may be loss of vascular tone resulting in vascular dilatation. The vessels cannot be adequately filled by the volume of blood and the consequence is hypotension and reduced tissue perfusion. Cardiac function is normal.

Clinical correlation

By definition a patient in shock has hypotension. There is also tachycardia produced by the sympathetic drive. Other symptoms and signs vary according to the aetiology and can be useful in determining the cause of shock clinically.

Hypovolaemic and cardiogenic shock. Both are associated with a cold, pale skin owing to vasoconstriction, and a weak, thready pulse owing to reduced cardiac output. However, cardiogenic shock will also be associated with features of systemic and/or pulmonary congestion, such as jugular venous distension and rales on auscultation.

Septic shock. Patients have warm peripheries, at least initially, from vasodilatation. As septic shock enters the hypodynamic phase, the circulation fails, and the skin becomes cold and clammy. Acute respiratory distress syndrome is a common complication of septic shock and reflects alveolar damage from hypoxia and inflammatory mediators.

Neurogenic shock. Typical presentation is with warm peripheries and hypotension plus evidence of spinal or cerebral injury.

Anaphylactic shock. Diagnosis is based on sudden cardiovascular collapse following exposure to the responsible antigen.

Other features are common to shock irrespective of the aetiology.

Urine output. This is reduced in shocked patients. Initially, this represents retention of salt and water to increase the circulating volume. However, if the kidneys suffer hypoxic damage, acute tubular necrosis occurs and kidney function fails, reducing the urine output further. This is the pathophysiological rationale behind monitoring urine output in patients with shock.

Cerebral function. Because neurons are particularly sensitive to hypoxia, an altered mental status becomes quickly evident as cerebral perfusion falls.

Acidosis. Persistent tissue hypoxia causes metabolic lactic acidosis, which causes arteriolar dilatation, decreased vascular resistance, and a further decrease in blood pressure.

Multiple organ dysfunction syndrome (MODS). As shock progresses, the patient develops multiorgan failure. MODS is defined as the presence of altered organ function in an acutely ill patient such that homeostasis cannot be maintained without intervention. In the case of septic shock, circulating inflammatory mediators compound the tissue damage. Common manifestations of MODS in shock are:

- **heart**: systolic and/or diastolic dysfunction, arrhythmia, myocardial ischaemia
- **central nervous system**: encephalopathy, infarction
- **kidneys**: prerenal failure, acute tubular necrosis
- **lungs**: acute respiratory distress syndrome
- **stomach, intestines**: erosive gastritis, ileus, infarction
- **liver**: ischaemic failure, cholestasis
- **gallbladder**: acalculous cholecystitis
- **pancreas**: acute pancreatitis
- **blood**: thrombocytopenia, DIC
- **immune system**: immunosuppression.

Eventually, there may be such severe organ damage that the shock becomes irreversible (**refractory shock**), and death becomes inevitable despite treatment.

14. Healing of wounds and fractures

Questions
- What are the processes involved in wound and fracture healing?
- What factors may interfere with efficient wound and fracture healing?

Wound healing

Healing of wounds involves inflammation, granulation tissue formation and fibrosis. The process is controlled by a complex network of cell–cell and cell–matrix interactions. Inflammatory cells are required to fight infection, especially in contaminated wounds. Phagocytes remove necrotic tissue and blood clot and also attempt to digest particles of foreign material contaminating the wound (the last is characterized histologically by foreign body giant cells). Granulation tissue revascularizes the damaged tissue, and the deposition of collagen and other matrix materials leads to the formation of a scar (Ch. 7).

If there has been a breach in an epithelial surface, epithelial cells from the edge of the wound grow over the granulation tissue, reepithelializing the damaged area (Fig. 3.14.1). This process is also controlled by a complex series of cell–cell and cell–matrix interactions.

Factors inhibiting wound healing

There are a number of factors that can inhibit wound healing.

Persistent infection. The inflammation associated with defence against pathogens inhibits healing.

Presence of a foreign body. A foreign body provides a site where bacteria may be protected from the host defence mechanisms, because the foreign material inhibits access of antibodies and inflammatory cells. Furthermore, if the foreign body is indigestible, granulation tissue cannot organize it. Therefore, foreign bodies can be said to act as a 'sanctuary site' for bacteria.

Stasis. Contaminating bacteria may be removed by the flow of secretions and excretions (e.g. tears and urine). If stasis (i.e. lack of flow) of a fluid occurs, contaminating bacteria can multiply within it. For example, in urinary outflow obstruction associated with incomplete emptying of the bladder, any bacteria that manage to ascend the urethra into the bladder have a chance to multiply in the urine and cause urinary tract infection.

Poor blood supply. Blood is required to bring the cells involved in healing to the site and provide oxygen for their high metabolic demands. For these reasons, wounds to the highly vascularized head and neck region tend to heal quickly whereas wounds to the poorly perfused shins and ankles often heal slowly.

Deficiency of substances required for collagen synthesis. Vitamin C and zinc, for example, are required for collagen production. Wounds in patients deficient in these substances heal slowly and are likely to break down, if they heal at all.

Immunodeficiency. The immune system may be depressed by acquired disease processes such as acquired immunodeficiency syndrome (AIDS), malnutrition and extremes of age, or by inherited immune deficiencies such as X-linked agammaglobulinaemia. It may also be depressed therapeutically by drugs (e.g. steroids and other immunosuppressants) or by radiotherapy. The excess production of steroid hormones in Cushing's syndrome has a similar effect. Any of these factors can inhibit healing.

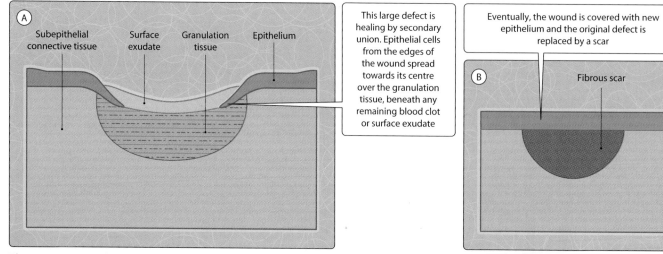

A

| Subepithelial connective tissue | Surface exudate | Granulation tissue | Epithelium |

This large defect is healing by secondary union. Epithelial cells from the edges of the wound spread towards its centre over the granulation tissue, beneath any remaining blood clot or surface exudate

Eventually, the wound is covered with new epithelium and the original defect is replaced by a scar

B   Fibrous scar

Fig. 3.14.1 Re-epithelialization in a wound.

Fracture healing

Bones break as a result of a sudden trauma that exceeds the strength of the bone. If the bone is abnormal, the degree of trauma required may be relatively slight, for example in bones weakened by osteoporosis or the presence of a neoplasm. Fractures through abnormal bone are called **pathological fractures.**

Another type of fracture is the **stress (fatigue) fracture.** In these injuries, it is not a single episode of major trauma but repeated episodes of minor trauma that result in the bone breaking. This phenomenon is familiar to engineers because the molecular structure of metals can be rearranged in response to repeated stress, allowing a crack to develop and failure of a metal that is subjected to repeated stresses, such as engine parts. In medicine, stress fractures are most commonly observed after prolonged marching, training for sport or long-distance running, and usually occur in the tibia, fibula or metatarsals.

Fracture healing involves many of the processes described above (Fig. 3.14.2). The first event is the formation of a haematoma of bleeding from ruptured vessels. There will also be fragments of devitalized bone and damaged soft tissue that will become necrotic. The haematoma and necrotic material are organized by granulation tissue. This granulation tissue contains osteoblasts, which produce new bone of woven type. The result is that the fractured ends are linked by a callus of woven bone that acts as a splint. In most cases, cartilage is also formed in the callus; it is then converted into bone.

Remodelling of the callus occurs as the healing process continues; excess callus is resorbed and the new bone is transformed from woven type to lamellar type. The lamellar bone itself is gradually remodelled according to the direction of mechanical stress experienced by the bone.

Any of the factors that impair healing in general can inhibit fracture healing. However, there are also several factors specific to bony injury that can interfere with fracture healing:

- an excess of haematoma, dead bone or necrotic tissue
- soft tissue interposed between the fractured ends
- movement of the fractured ends relative to each other, particularly rotatory or shearing movement that severs the capillaries in the developing granulation tissue
- severe misalignment
- impaired blood supply to one of the fragments
- preexisting bone disease.

These factors tend to promote **fibrous union:** the bone ends become linked by fibrous tissue rather than bone. This fibrous tissue ossifies slowly. As a result, the fracture takes an excessive time to heal and the term used is **delayed union.** If there is complete failure of bony union the term **non-union** is used. Occasionally, if movement between the ends is severe and prolonged, a synovial joint develops in the fibrous tissue (a false joint or pseudarthrosis). **Mal-union** implies deformity of the healed fracture and results from imperfect alignment of the fragments during the healing process.

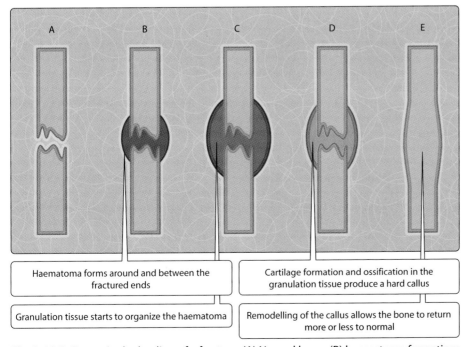

| Haematoma forms around and between the fractured ends | Cartilage formation and ossification in the granulation tissue produce a hard callus |
| Granulation tissue starts to organize the haematoma | Remodelling of the callus allows the bone to return more or less to normal |

Fig. 3.14.2 Stages in the healing of a fracture. (A) Normal bone; (B) haematoma formation; (C) granulation; (D) formation of a hard callus; (E) remodelling of the callus.

15. Vasculitis

Questions
- What are the pathological mechanisms involved in the development of vasculitis?
- What are the clinical manifestations of vasculitis?

Blood vessels play an important part in all inflammatory conditions but there are a number of disorders in which the vessels are the primary site of the inflammatory process, and the term vasculitis is used specifically for these. The vasculitides are classified according to the size of vessel involved (Fig. 3.15.1), the clinicopathological features of the disease and whether there is evidence of antineutrophil cytoplasmic antibodies (ANCA). There is considerable overlap among the diagnostic entities, and classification depends on many factors, including patient age, clinical symptoms and signs, ANCA status and pathological changes in biopsies.

Antineutrophil cytoplasmic antibodies

The ANCAs are antibodies for antigens in neutrophil lysosomes. There are two main varieties: p-ANCA and c-ANCA, named for their pattern on immunofluorescence (perinuclear and cytoplasmic, respectively). It has been discovered that p-ANCA mainly reacts with myeloperoxidase whereas c-ANCA mainly reacts with proteinase 3, so modern laboratory methods test for these antibodies specifically. Positivity for ANCA is associated with microscopic polyangiitis, Churg–Strauss syndrome and Wegener granulomatosis. In particular, a positive c-ANCA is good evidence of Wegener granulomatosis.

Pathogenesis of vasculitis

The pathological mechanisms underlying the vasculitis syndromes are only partially understood. There seem to be four main types of process.

Deposition of immune complexes in the walls of vessels. This process occurs in conditions of relative antigen excess, and is seen in polyarteritis nodosa (often in patients with hepatitis B or C) and Henoch–Schönlein purpura. The immune complexes initiate inflammation.

Antiendothelial antibodies. In some vasculitides, for example Kawasaki disease and possibly Buerger disease (thromboangiitis obliterans), there is evidence that autoantibodies to endothelial cells are responsible.

ANCA. There is some evidence that ANCA may have a pathogenic role in those conditions in which it is found (i.e. microscopic polyangiitis, Churg–Strauss syndrome and Wegener granulomatosis). If ANCA interacts with neutrophils it activates them, causing the neutrophils to degranulate, produce reactive oxygen species and secrete pro-inflammatory cytokines.

Granulomatous inflammation. A variety of immune responses causes T-cells and macrophages to cooperate in the production of granulomas. This process is seen in giant cell arteritis, Takayasu arteritis, Churg–Strauss syndrome and Wegener granulomatosis.

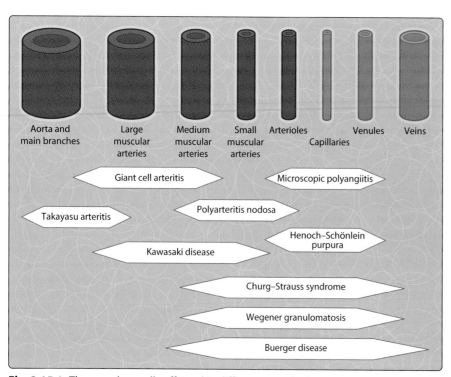

Fig. 3.15.1 The vessels usually affected in different vasculitides.

Pathology of vasculitis

In most forms of vasculitis an infiltrate of acute and chronic inflammatory cells is present in the wall of the vessel and the adjacent tissues. Giant cell arteritis and Takayasu arteritis characteristically also have multinucleated giant cells. It is often possible to demonstrate deposits of antibodies and complement in vessel walls in those cases that are caused by immune mechanisms. Common to all types is that the inflammation often heals by fibrosis, giving a fibrous scar. Fibrinoid necrosis of the vessel wall is common in some types of vasculitis, for example polyarteritis nodosa and Kawasaki disease. It weakens the wall and can be associated with dilation of the affected vessel (aneurysm formation).

Granulomatous inflammation with necrosis is typical of Wegener granulomatosis and Churg–Strauss syndrome; the latter shows large numbers of eosinophils in the inflammatory infiltrate. In microscopic polyangiitis, large numbers of fragmented neutrophils are usually found, giving this condition its alternative name of leukocytoclastic vasculitis.

Three mechanisms cause most of the effects of vasculitis: obstruction by thrombosis or fibrosis causes ischaemia, damaged vessels allow haemorrhage, and inflammation has general systemic effects such as fever and malaise. The clinical features will depend on the vessels affected (Table 3.15.1).

Table 3.15.1 CLINICAL FEATURES OF SOME OF THE VASCULITIS SYNDROMES

Vasculitis	Typical individuals affected	Common clinical manifestations	Comments
Giant cell (temporal) arteritis	Adults over 50 years	Fever; weight loss; headache; facial pain; tenderness of temporal artery; ocular symptoms if ophthalmic artery involved (can cause blindness)	Often involves temporal artery (hence temporal arteritis); temporal artery biopsy is a diagnostic test
Polyarteritis nodosa	Young adults typically, but wide age range with children and elderly also affected	Fever; weight loss; localized symptoms very variable and depend on vessels affected (e.g. hypertension; abdominal pain; peripheral neuritis; muscle pains; renal failure)	The inflammation typically affects segments of arteries, causing lesions that are firm and nodular to palpation, hence its name
Henoch–Schönlein purpura	Children	Palpable purpura of buttocks and lower limbs; gastrointestinal symptoms; arthritis; glomerulonephritis	Immune complex mediated; immune complexes usually contain IgA
Kawasaki disease	Infants and children.	Acute illness with fever, skin rash, inflammation of mouth and conjunctiva, enlarged cervical nodes; often affects coronary arteries, causing acute coronary syndrome or coronary artery aneurysm (which can rupture)	Also called mucocutaneous lymph node syndrome
Takayasu arteritis	Females under 40 years	Fever; weight loss; neurological symptoms and blindness; hypertension from renal artery narrowing; pulmonary hypertension from pulmonary artery involvement	Alternative name of pulseless disease derives from weakening of upper limb pulses
Microscopic polyangiitis (leukocytoclastic vasculitis, hypersensitivity vasculitis)	Wide age range	Purpuric skin rash; glomerulonephritis; arthritis; bowel pain; pulmonary capillaritis with haemoptysis; may be part of other autoimmune conditions, e.g. systemic lupus erthrymatosus, rheumatoid arthritis, Sjögren syndrome	Often ANCA positive
Churg–Strauss syndrome (allergic granulomatosis and angiitis)	Individuals with atopy, asthma, allergic rhinitis	Lung, nerve and upper respiratory tract usually involved; eosinophilia characteristic	Often ANCA positive
Wegener granulomatosis	Adults	Fever; weight loss; many organs can be involved, especially upper respiratory tract, lung and kidney	c-ANCA positive in over 90%
Buerger disease (thromboangiitis obliterans)	Young or middle-aged adults; positive smoking history	Ischaemia of extremities; inflammation may spread to adjacent nerves causing severe pain	Strong association with smoking

ANCA, antineutrophil cytoplasmic antibodies.

16. Host defence

Questions
- What are the major components of the immune system?
- What are the mechanisms by which cells and tissues are protected against injurious agents?
- What is a clinical example of a disease resulting from impaired host defence?

The body is under continual threat from injury from a wide range of causes (Ch. 9). A wide range of mechanisms exists to counter these: behavioural changes, physical barriers and the presence of an immune system. **Innate immunity** is the first line of defence; it is present at birth and has no specificity or memory and comprises physicochemical barriers, humoral components (e.g. complement) and cells (e.g. mast cells). **Acquired immunity** describes the adaptive responses acquired during development through exposure (Ch. 17).

Behavioural protective mechanisms

Humans have developed the ability to influence their environment to an extraordinary degree. These generally allow the avoidance of extremes of temperature and potentially the minimization of the risk of trauma. Protective reflexes include the cough reflex and the blink reflex. Therefore, individuals who are unable to cough because of neurological disease or physical disease involving the chest or abdomen are especially prone to the development of pneumonia. Conditions that impair the ability to swallow will lead to an increased risk of aspiration of gastric contents and pneumonia. Pneumonia is, therefore, a very common terminal condition in elderly patients or those with severe coexistent diseases such as severe strokes or advanced malignancy (Ch. 42).

Physical barriers to infection

The skin and the epithelia lining the hollow viscera provide a physical barrier. The skin is a complex collection of tissues that, when intact, protects the body from a wide range of physical and microbial threats (Fig. 3.16.1):

- **stratified squamous epithelium** provides a tough multilayered physical defence against trauma, temperature excesses and microorganisms in the surface skin, the oesophagus and the anal canal
- **hairs** can erect to provide an extended barrier to the skin and additional insulation against low temperatures
- **sweat glands** allow loss of heat from body in high temperatures (intrinsic or extrinsic)

The lining of the hollow viscera have specific protective devices:

- the **mucosal lining** itself has a partly defensive role

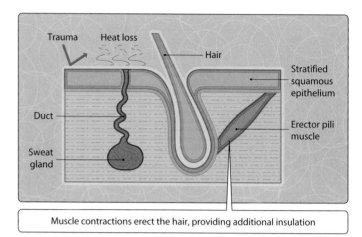

Fig. 3.16.1 The skin provides an initial barrier against physical and microbial threats.

- the **mucociliary escalator** established by cilia and mucus in the respiratory tract allows the removal of particles, including microorganisms, from the airways
- **mucus** throughout the gastrointestinal tract provides lubrication, protects against sharp materials, and provides a pH gradient between the contents and the cells lining the tract; hydrochloric acid in the stomach kills microorganisms (Fig. 3.16.2).

It is, therefore, essential that mechanisms exist for the rapid repair of defects within the skin or mucosal surfaces in order to preserve the integrity of these barriers, and continuous turnover of epithelial cells is essential. The good blood supply throughout facilitates the high cell turnover and also removes undesirable molecules, for example removal of excess hydrogen ions from the lamina propria of the stomach.

Other barrier defences include tears bathing the conjunctivae and salivary glands producing saliva to cleanse the oral cavity.

The immune system

A correctly functioning immune system is clearly essential for the minimization of the risk of tissue injury through infection. The immune system comprises a complex network of many different cell types that work together to provide a defence against microorganisms that gain access to the body. Some components of the immune system are also able to recognize and destroy early neoplastic cells, thereby offering surveillance for the development of neoplasia. Immunoreactive cells are present within the bone marrow and blood as well as within most solid tissues. The two major arms of the immune system are those providing **cellular immunity** and **humoral immunity**. Acute and chronic inflammation (Chs 3–6) occurs as a result of various stimuli (Chs 8 and 9) and

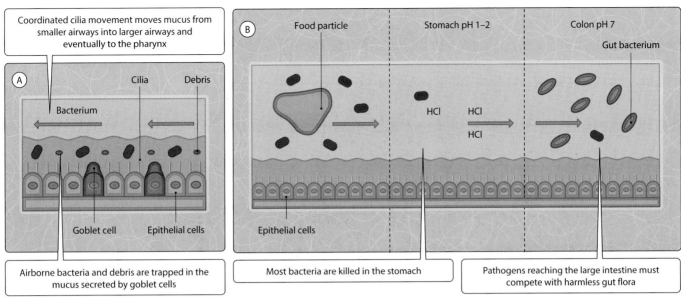

Fig. 3.16.2 Mucosal barriers to infection.

involves many of these cell types, both in non-specific reactions to tissue injury and *specific* reactions to certain microorganisms and other proteins; the latter is termed a true 'immune' reaction. A complex range of special interactions occurs between cells making up the immune system in order to orchestrate a coherent specific immune reaction. The immune system can cause damage to the body if inappropriate reactions occur (see Ch. 45).

Components of the immune system

The major cellular components of the immune system are listed in Table 3.16.1. These immunoreactive cells are derived from the bone marrow and are present within the blood as well as within tissues with a major role in immunity (e.g. lymph nodes, spleen) and many other tissues with other main functions; the numbers of immunoreactive cells within these other organs is highly variable and depends upon the organ's function and the anatomical relationship of the organ to the external environment. For example, the intestine is a critical interface between the environment and the body, contains large numbers of commensal bacteria (i.e. bacteria living normally within the lumen of the intestine and not associated, at least in healthy individuals, with the development of infection) and contains large numbers of lymphocytes, plasma cells and macrophages mainly within the lamina propria of the mucosa and in areas in very close relationship to the lining epithelium.

Table 3.16.1 COMPOSITION OF THE IMMUNE SYSTEM

Cell type	Function
Neutrophils	Acute inflammation: degranulation and microbial killing
Eosinophils	Allergic and parasitic conditions; role uncertain
Lymphocytes B (10–20%)[a] T (60-70%)[a] Plasma cells Natural killer cells (10–15%)[a]	Humoral immunity Cellular immunity Antibody production Lysis of virally infected cells and tumour cells
Macrophages	Phagocytosis (especially of opsonized antigens); antigen presentation; cytokine production; immunosurveillance for tumour cells
Dendritic cells and Langerhans' cells	Antigen presentation (via Fc receptors, which trap antigen-antibody immune complexes)[b]

[a]*Proportion of the total number of lymphocytes.*
[b]*Fc receptors bind to the Fc region of antibody molecules.*

17. Basic immunology

Questions
- What are the functions of the immune system?
- What is cellular and humoral immunity?
- How does the immune system carry out its functions?

Cellular immunity

Cellular immunity is achieved by immunoreactive cells that directly destroy cells tagged for destruction. Essentially there are two types of such cell: cells that have become infected (e.g. by viruses) or, in certain situations, neoplastic cells and cells that have phagocytosed foreign antigen. Cells are tagged by the production on their cell surface of antigen fragments from the 'invader' attached to molecules known as the major histocompatibility complex (MHC; called the human leukocyte antigen (HLA) system in humans). The component chains making up a class I or II molecule are known as HLA antigens.

Cells that have become infected can be recognized by a subset of T-lymphocytes termed **cytotoxic lymphocytes** via presentation of processed viral antigens attached to MHC class I molecules on the surface of the infected cells, which are killed directly. Foreign antigen can be phagocytosed by **antigen-presenting cells** such as macrophages, which process the antigens before expressing modified fragments on the surface of their cytoplasmic membrane attached to class II molecules. Killing of these cells by cytotoxic T-lymphocytes is stimulated by interactions with **helper T-lymphocytes**, which themselves can recognize foreign antigens presented to them by MHC class II molecules on the surface of antigen-presenting cells and in association with the CD4 T-cell receptor. Two subsets of helper T-lymphocytes exist; Th1 cells secrete cytokines that help to induce cellular immunity (i.e. via the stimulation of CD8 T-lymphocytes) while Th2 cells secrete cytokines that promote humoral immunity. Cytotoxic T-lymphocytes recognize virally infected cells by class I molecules with antigen fragments on the surface of the infected cells in association with the CD8 T-cell receptor (Fig. 3.17.1).

Polymorphism within genes encoding the MHC

The genes encoding the HLA molecules are extremely polymorphic (i.e. have many potential forms) and this polymorphism particularly affects the amino acid sequences within the antigen-binding groove, resulting in subtle alterations in shape and, therefore, small differences in the efficiency of antigen presentation. This leads to small interindividual differences in modulation of the immune response to a wide range of antigens and to varying susceptibility to a range of diseases, both neoplastic and non-neoplastic, in which development and progression is affected by the immune system (e.g. autoimmune diseases; Ch. 18).

Development of B- and T-lymphocytes

All lymphocytes derive from multipotential stem cells within bone marrow. Immature T-lymphocytes that have not been exposed to any antigens (*naive* T-lymphocytes) travel to the thymus where huge diversity in their T-cell receptors is generated via genetic rearrangements within the genes encoding the T-cell receptors. This resulting population can potentially recognize and, therefore, respond to a very large range of antigens. T-lymphocytes found to react to self-antigens are then destroyed in the thymus as one of several mechanisms that prevent the body being damaged by its own immune system (i.e. the induction of **tolerance**). The remaining T-lymphocytes then populate lymphoid tissues such as the lymph nodes and spleen and are ready to encounter foreign antigens.

Immature B-lymphocytes undergo maturation, including rearrangements of the genes encoding immunoglobulin heavy chains, within the lymph nodes and spleen, without travelling first to the thymus. In a manner *analogous* to the development of immunoreactive T-lymphocytes, this also produces a population of cells that can potentially recognize and, therefore, respond to a very large range of antigens.

Stimulation of B- and T-lymphocytes leads to the production of antibodies and cytotoxic T-lymphocytes but *also* leads to the production of **memory** B- and T-lymphocytes, which remain dormant within lymphoid tissues but are ready to promote an effective immune response should the individual encounter the same antigen in the future.

Antigen-presenting cells

Many cells can process antigens and present them on their cytoplasmic membrane for recognition by other immunoreactive cells. The most common antigen-presenting cell is the macrophage and related cells of similar lineage. Some antigen-presenting cells possess long cytoplasmic processes (e.g. dendritic cells within lymphoid tissue, Langerhans' cells within the skin) and these increase the efficiency of antigen presentation. Follicular dendritic cells are found within the germinal centres of lymphoid aggregates and trap antigens bound to antibody via an Fc receptor for the antibody that is present on the surface of the follicular dendritic cell; this provides a mechanism for augmenting immunological memory. B-lymphocytes may also act as antigen-presenting cells in certain situations.

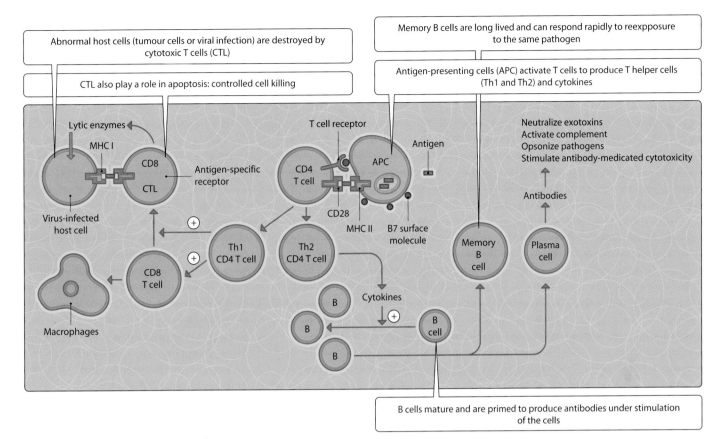

Fig. 3.17.1 Immune responses to infection.

Natural killer cells

Many interactions between immunoreactive cells and antigens occur via HLA molecule-mediated mechanisms (HLA-restricted; i.e. binding of target cell class I or class II molecules, each enclosing antigenic peptides, to T-cell receptors *and* to CD8 and CD4 molecules, respectively, on CD8 and CD4 T-lymphocytes) and, therefore, occur in association with very accurate recognition of antigens by specific immunoreactive cells. However, a subset of immunoreactive cells termed natural killer cells is able to destroy other cells *without* the requirement for previous sensitization and HLA-mediated recognition. Natural killer cells are a subset of lymphocytes that do *not* bear the CD3 molecule and which appear particularly important for lysis of virally infected cells and tumour cells. Natural killer cells bear surface Fc receptors that bind to antibodies, allowing antibody-mediated cellular cytotoxicity (ADCC) to occur. These cells also bear surface stimulatory receptors that bind to poorly defined molecules on target cells and lead to target cell killing. Although lysis mediated by natural killer cells does not depend upon HLA-restricted target cell binding, these cells do bear surface receptors for class I molecules, thus allowing binding to and recognition of normal self-cells; this binding process overrides the stimulatory receptors and, therefore, prevents lysis of normal self-cells.

Humoral immunity

The humoral system provides defence against infection through the production of antibodies, which act by:

- neutralization of microorganisms (especially bacteria and fungi) and toxins
- opsonization
- activation of complement
- ADCC
- mast cell degranulation (IgE)
- signal transduction within immunoreactive cells.

Opsonization is a process whereby foreign antigens become coated with antibody and this then promotes phagocytosis of the coated antigen by cells such as macrophages. Antibodies are produced by plasma cells, which are derived from activated B-lymphocytes. B-lymphocytes recognize and are stimulated by foreign antigens that bind to immunoglobulin molecules on their cytoplasmic membrane surface and are also stimulated to differentiate into plasma cells via interactions with helper T-lymphocytes.

The **complement cascade** refers to a group of soluble proteins within the blood that can become activated by a range of stimuli, which then results in the production of several active proteins with specific functions in the promotion of an immune response (Ch. 8).

18. Autoimmune disease

Questions
- How is immune-mediated damage to an individual's own tissues avoided?
- Which diseases can result from failure of these mechanisms?

The immune system is closely regulated to minimize the risk of self-antigens being recognized as foreign, leading to immune-mediated damage to an individual's own cells and tissues. This regulation occurs by mechanisms that induce **immune tolerance** (Fig. 3.18.1). Suppressor CD8 T cells can also inhibit the immune response, in part by releasing inhibitory cytokines (e.g. IL-10). Autoimmune diseases develop when one or more of these protective mechanisms fails or is bypassed.

Mechanisms of autoimmune disease development

Infective agents
Some infectious agents may possess epitopes (i.e. antigenic components) that are sufficiently similar to self-antigens to generate cross-reactivity during the immune response (molecular mimicry). In rheumatic fever, cross-reactivity occurs between streptococcal antigens (commonly associated with pharyngeal infection) and self-antigens, leading to autoimmune-mediated inflammation at several sites within the body. This inflammation gives the classical multisystem clinical features of acute rheumatic fever (fleeting arthritis, endocarditis and myocarditis). This mechanism may also be important in the development of type 1 diabetes mellitus, with cross-reactivity occurring between coxsackievirus and beta cell antigens.

The immune response to some infective agents may be associated with **polyclonal reactivation** of circulating autoreactive lymphocytes that have previously been inactivated via the clonal inactivation mechanism (Fig. 3.18.1). This, in turn, can promote the development of autoimmune disease.

Imbalance between helper and suppressor T cells
It is possible that a relative excess of helper T-lymphocyte function or a deficiency of suppressor T-lymphocyte function may induce autoimmune responses.

Exposure of sequestered self-antigens
Trauma or infection may expose self-antigens to the immune system that normally exists in 'privileged sites' to which immunoreactive cells do not gain access. For example, inflammatory and/or traumatic injury to one eye can result in the exposure of ocular antigens and to autoimmune damage within both eyes.

The role of immunogenetics
Correct functioning of the immune system is reliant upon complex interactions between immunoreactive cells and their targets. These interactions involve molecules present on the surfaces of cells, many of which are transmembrane in nature and, therefore, may also interact with intracytoplasmic components. Many of the genes encoding molecules such as the HLA family and cytokines (or their promoter regions) are highly polymorphic (meaning that one or more variants of the genes exist) and these polymorphisms may alter the detailed structure of the molecules (e.g. the antigen-binding groove of HLA molecules) or possibly the level of expression of molecules (e.g. cytokines). These changes can modulate immune responses, leading to

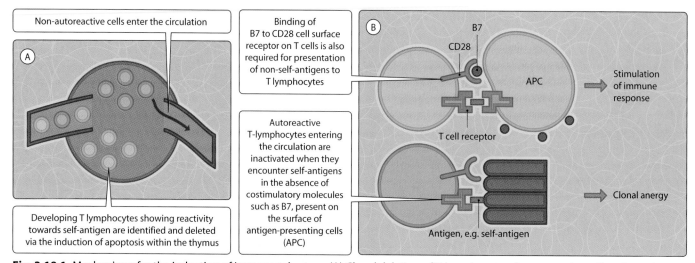

Fig. 3.18.1 Mechanisms for the induction of immune tolerance. (A) Clonal deletion of T-lymphocytes that recognize self-antigens (may also occur for B-cells but this is of less importance); (B) clonal anergy.

interindividual differences in the response to antigens and the risk of development of forms of aberrant immune response such as those characterizing autoimmune disease. Individuals possessing certain HLA genetic polymorphisms are at increased risk of developing particular autoimmune diseases (Table 3.18.1).

The spectrum of autoimmune disease

Autoimmune diseases may primarily affect one tissue type or organ or may show multisystem involvement. Patients with one form of autoimmune disease are often at risk of development of further autoimmune diseases since they possess a genetic constitution that predisposes them to this spectrum of conditions. For example, patients with type 1 diabetes mellitus are at increased risk of developing coeliac disease. Clinical overlap can also occur between some of these diseases such that the clinical and pathological features as present in a particular patient may be part of the spectrum usually seen in more than one autoimmune disease; this occurs, for example, in connective tissue diseases and between the autoimmune conditions affecting the liver.

The pathology of autoimmune disease

Autoimmune diseases are usually characterized by a combination of inflammation (usually chronic) and tissue damage; the latter may result in tissue scarring and/or loss of cellular/organ function. Autoimmune diseases resulting in damage to highly specific cell types may result in no macroscopically identifiable abnormality. For example, type 1 diabetes mellitus results from autoimmune destruction of insulin-producing beta cells within the pancreatic islets; this would be identifiable using immunohistochemistry and microscopy of pancreatic tissue but the pancreas would appear normal to the naked eye. In contrast, rheumatoid disease is a multisystem disorder characterized, when advanced, by obvious deformities of affected joints (e.g. those within the hand) as well as cutaneous nodules, pericarditis and pulmonary fibrosis (Chs 51, 52 and 60).

Clinical course of autoimmune diseases

The clinical features of autoimmune disease are highly varied and depend upon the tissues/organs targeted by the process. They can be divided into two groups:

- **organ/tissue-specific disorders**: type 1 diabetes mellitus (pancreas: islet beta cells), autoimmune haemolytic anaemia (red blood cells), autoimmune thrombocytopoenic purpura (platelets), Graves' disease (thyroid: thyroid-stimulating hormone receptors), pernicious anaemia (stomach: parietal cells), coeliac disease (small intestine: mucosa), autoimmune hepatitis (liver: hepatocytes), autoimmune cholangiopathy, primary biliary cirrhosis and primary sclerosing cholangitis (liver: bile ducts), scleroderma (skin) and myasthenia gravis (neuromuscular junctions)
- **multisystem disorders**: rheumatic fever, connective tissue diseases (e.g. rheumatoid arthritis, systemic lupus erythematosus, systemic sclerosis and CREST syndrome (a 'limited' form of scleroderma characterized by: calcinosis, Raynaud's phenomenon, oesophageal dysmotility, sclerodactyly and telangiectasia).

Autoimmune diseases are chronic, commonly slowly progressive and often 'incurable'. Because most tissues have reserve capacity, diseases may not become clinically evident until most of the targeted cell type has been destroyed (e.g. diabetes mellitus). Others may present at a relatively earlier stage, for example scleroderma, and still others may enter remission if a triggering stimulus is removed (e.g. coeliac disease after introduction of a gluten-free diet). The progression of some autoimmune diseases may be slowed with immunosuppressive therapy (e.g. steroids, azathioprine). If a particular cell type is destroyed, then replacement therapy is usually required (e.g. insulin treatment in type I diabetes mellitus, corticosteroid replacement in Addison's disease). Transplantation of cells (e.g. beta islet cells) may be a therapeutic approach but one difficulty will be the procurement of sufficient replacement cells; stem cell research may enable fully differentiated (i.e. mature and functional) replacement cells to be created for this and other purposes.

Table 3.18.1 ASSOCIATIONS BETWEEN HLA ALLELES AND AUTOIMMUNE DISEASES

Disease	Associated HLA locus/allele	Relative risk[a]
Coeliac disease	DQ2	250
Ankylosing spondylitis	B27	> 150
Reactive disease	B27	> 40
Type 1 diabetes mellitus[b]	DQ8	14
	DQ6	0.02
Multiple sclerosis	DR2, DQ6	12
Rheumatoid arthritis	DR4	9
Haemochromatosis	A3	6
Addison's disease	DR3	5
Graves' disease	DR3	4
Myasthenia gravis	DR3	2

[a]Relative risk measures frequently of the disease in question in individuals with an HLA locus allele compared with those not carrying the allele.
[b]Complex HLA associations occur.

19. Immunodeficiency

Questions
- What is immunodeficiency?
- How can immunodeficiency occur?
- What clinical problems can immunodeficiency create?

Immunodeficiency refers to a state in which the immune system does not work with full efficiency, leading primarily to an increased risk of infections. Since the immune system also detects and destroys some tumour cells, patients with immunodeficiency may also be at increased risk of neoplasia. For example, patients on long-term immunosuppression following a solid organ transplant such as a kidney are at increased risk of developing cutaneous squamous cell carcinoma and Epstein–Barr virus-driven lymphoproliferative disorder (a virally triggered proliferation of immature lymphoid cells that behaves in a similar way to lymphoma).

Causes of immunodeficiency

There are many reasons why immunodeficiency may occur. Some of these are congenital (primary) and, therefore, affect neonates and children while others may be acquired (secondary) during childhood or adulthood.

Primary causes:

- common variable immunodeficiency
- severe combined immunodeficiency
- chronic granulomatous disease
- specific immunoglobulin deficiencies.

Secondary causes:

- malnutrition
- serious systemic disease: cancer, renal disease, conditions resulting in bone marrow destruction or interference with the normal function of marrow (e.g. leukaemia)
- iatrogenic: chemotherapy, post-transplant anti-rejection drugs, immunosuppressive drugs for chronic inflammatory conditions (e.g. connective tissue diseases, inflammatory bowel disease)
- infective: HIV infection
- splenectomy: traumatic or secondary, for example to sickle cell disease.

Iatrogenic causes of immunodeficiency are important and relatively common, especially with the increasing range of chemotherapeutic drugs available for neoplasia, immunosuppressive therapies for chronic inflammatory diseases, and increasing numbers of organ transplants.

Primary immunodeficiency

Primary immunodeficiencies vary in clinical severity from conditions that, if untreated, are incompatible with life (e.g. severe combined immunodeficiency) to conditions that may not require specific treatment (e.g. common variable immunodeficiency). They may predominantly affect one component of the immune system (e.g. hypogammaglobulinaemia, in which one or more class of antibody may be affected, or chronic granulomatous disease, in which the ability to kill phagocytosed microorganisms such as bacteria is impaired) or may affect the functioning of both the humoral and cellular arms of the immune system (e.g. severe combined immunodeficiency). However, almost all forms will be associated with increased risk of infections. Accurate diagnosis of an immunodeficiency syndrome usually requires detailed specialist testing of the components of the immune system. However, some are associated with characteristic changes within tissue biopsies. For example, common variable immunodeficiency is often associated with the presence of *Giardia lamblia* parasites on duodenal biopsy. The more serious forms of primary immunodeficiency may be treatable by bone marrow transplantation. Less severe types (e.g. hypogammaglobulinaemia) may only be diagnosed as a result of specific investigations performed to investigate recurrent infections such as pneumonia.

Secondary immunodeficiency

There are numerous causes of secondary immunodeficiency, some of which relate to specific defects while others occur as a result of generalized disease processes. The importance of the latter in clinical medicine is that elderly patients or those with malnutrition or serious conditions such as cancer are at increased risk of the development of infection *even in the absence of an additional more specific risk factor*.

HIV infection

HIV infection and its clinical outcome, AIDS, is an increasing problem worldwide (currently around 40 million people are believed to be infected with HIV worldwide). Although new therapies have very significantly slowed the progression of the disease in developed countries, untreated HIV infection is a leading cause of death in regions such as sub-Saharan Africa. The disease is endemic in Africa but in other parts of the world it occurs particularly within risk groups characterized by the transfer of body fluids.

Epidemiology of HIV infection

The two largest risk groups are homosexual contact and intravenous drug usage. Other risk groups include heterosexual contact, vertical transmission (i.e. mother to child, which occurs in up to 30% of those at risk), blood product recipients (non-haemophiliac) and haemophilia treatment (the last two within healthcare systems in which screening of donors for evidence of HIV infection did not or does not occur).

Structure of the HIV virus

Like all viruses, HIV comprises nucleic acid with surrounding protein coats (Fig. 3.19.1). HIV is a retrovirus; this means that its nucleic acid is RNA and that, on infection of host cells, the reverse transcriptase enzyme produced by the virus enables DNA to be constructed using the viral RNA as a template. This DNA becomes incorporated into the host DNA during the process of viral replication.

Mechanisms and sequelae of HIV infection

The HIV virus infects host cells that bear the CD4 surface receptor; this includes CD4 T-lymphocytes (helper type) and macrophages. Infection of host cells is followed by viral replication and host cell lysis, releasing multiple copies of the virus. The consequent loss of CD4-carrying immunoreactive cells leads to the major clinical consequence of HIV infection: immunodefiency. This is why the clinical syndrome is termed an **acquired immunodeficiency**. The HIV virus is particularly adept at evading the host immune response via alteration of the characteristics of its surface proteins. Furthermore, alterations in the viral components that are targeted by treatments may lead to resistance to treatment by that drug and by other drugs of a similar type (see below). Coreceptors on the cell surface, chemokine receptors such as CCR5, are required as well as CD4 receptors for internalization of HIV. Interestingly, individuals possessing mutations of the CCR5-encoding gene appear to be resistant to disease progression in HIV infection and are likely to become long-term survivors.

The clinical features of HIV infection follow a fairly characteristic sequence. Infection is usually followed by an asymptomatic period of around 3 months; during this period host antibodies to the virus are not detectable but HIV proteins can be. Seroconversion (i.e. the development of an immune response to the virus) may be associated with a brief febrile illness (in 50–70%), which has non-specific flu-like symptoms. When antibodies to HIV are detectable, the individual may be termed HIV positive. The clinical course is then variable. Before modern treatments, an asymptomatic period of 10 years (on average) would occur during which there was a gradual but irreversible decline in peripheral CD4 T-lymphocyte count; eventually the cell number would fall below a critical level (200×10^6 cells/l). After this time, the patient would gradually develop one or more (often opportunistic) infections and/or neoplasms characteristic of AIDS (Table 3.19.1; see also the box in Ch. 42). However, with modern treatment regimens, the outlook for HIV-infected patients who can gain access to these drugs is vastly improved; the proportion of patients alive at 10 years after initial diagnosis is now approximately double the number of long-term survivors before modern antiviral therapy. The inability of many HIV-infected people to access these treatments in endemic areas currently leads to soaring death rates from infection; in endemic areas within Africa, advanced HIV infection is very commonly associated with tuberculosis.

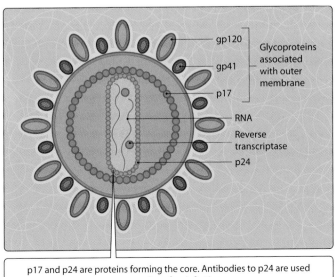

p17 and p24 are proteins forming the core. Antibodies to p24 are used as a marker of an infection

Fig. 3.19.1 The human immunodeficiency virus (HIV).

Table 3.19.1 INFECTIONS AND NEOPLASMS CHARACTERISTICALLY OCCURRING WITHIN AIDS

AIDS-associated disease	Example
Infections	
Mycobacteria	Tuberculosis and atypical mycobacterial infections: commonly clinically widespread e.g. miliary tuberculosis (Ch. 43)
Cytomegalovirus	Pneumonitis; retinitis
JC virus	Progressive multifocal leucoencephalopathy
Pneumocystis spp.	Pneumonia
Cryptococcus spp.	Meningitis
Toxoplasma sp.	Cerebral abscess
Neoplasms	
Kaposi's sarcoma[a]	Associated with herpes virus 8 infection
Cerebral lymphoma	Commonly fatal and so usually occurs as a clinically terminal event

[a]*May also (less commonly) develops outside HIV infection, usually on the lower extremities of elderly men.*

20. Definitions and nomenclature in neoplasia

Questions
- What is meant by the term neoplasia?
- What do neoplasms look like?
- How do we determine the clinical behaviour of neoplasms?

Neoplasia means new growth and is a broad term used to indicate a range of abnormal cellular proliferations. The term, therefore, includes established tumours (see below) and the cellular alterations that are recognized precursors to tumour development.

Tumour means 'swelling' and indicates the development of an abnormal population of cells. This change most commonly leads to the development of a mass (recognizable to the naked eye or only visible on histological examination, depending on its size) within preexisting non-neoplastic tissue, although this is not universally the case. For example, tumours of the bone marrow may replace normal marrow cells and lead to leukaemia without producing a recognizable mass.

Tumour development and differentiation
Most pathologists believe that tumours develop from a single primitive stem cell; these cells are themselves capable of development into one of several possible mature cell types. The histopathological appearances of tumour cells and tissues resemble normal tissues to a variable degree. The extent to which tumour tissues resemble normal tissues is termed the degree of differentiation of the tumour. Differentiation can only be assessed on microscopic examination of tumour tissue and is commonly subdivided into three categories (well, moderate and poor). Well-differentiated tumours show the greatest resemblance to normal tissues (e.g. an epithelial tumour forming glandular or ductal structures) while poorly differentiated tumours often comprise sheets of malignant cells showing little evidence of maturation into a particular tissue type. The growth pattern of a tumour is one component of the tumour characteristics that determine the tumour grade (see below).

Tumour type and nomenclature
Almost all tumours comprise cells showing differentiation towards one or more tissue type (e.g. epithelial), the name often reflecting the overall direction of differentiation in terms of tissue type and whether it is benign or malignant in nature:
- **epithelial**
  - benign: suffix *–oma*, e.g. adenoma, papilloma
  - malignant: suffix *carcinoma*, e.g. adenocarcinoma, squamous cell carcinoma, small cell carcinoma, undifferentiated carcinoma
- **mesenchymal**
  - benign: suffix *–oma*, e.g. leiomyoma, rhabdomyoma, fibroma, osteoma, chondroma, angioma
  - malignant: suffix *sarcoma*, e.g. leiomyosarcoma, rhabdomyosarcoma, fibrosarcoma, osteosarcoma, chondrosarcoma, angiosarcoma
- **lymphoid**
  - always malignant: suffix -*oma*, e.g. lymphoma
- **melanocytic**
  - always malignant: suffix -*oma*, e.g. melanoma.

The direction of differentiation of many tumours is more precisely defined by using a *prefix* within the tumour name. As examples, within epithelial tumours, *adeno* indicates glandular differentiation while *squamous* indicates squamous differentiation. Within mesenchymal tumours, *leio*, *rhabdo*, *angio*, *fibro*, *osteo* and *chondro* indicate smooth muscle, striated muscle, blood vessel, fibrous tissue, bone and cartilaginous differentiation, respectively.

Tumours often differentiate in a single direction but may develop several lines of differentiation, evidenced by a mixed growth pattern during microscopic examination. Examples of tumours showing dual differentiation are the mixed mullerian tumour of the uterus, and metaplastic carcinoma of the breast, which are aggressive cancers containing both epithelial (i.e. carcinomatous) and mesenchymal (i.e. sarcomatous) differentiation.

Tumour behaviour
Tumours behave biologically in a benign or malignant manner. Using a combination of clinical and pathological assessment, it is usually possible to predict the future behaviour of a tumour from its characteristics at or shortly after initial clinical presentation (see Ch. 23). Since the majority of these features are only reliably assessable during histopathological examination of the primary tumour or putative sites of metastasis, the pathologist is a key figure in the prediction of the biological behaviour of tumours. The most reliable features indicating that a tumour is malignant are a primary tumour with a poorly defined edge, invasion rather than compression of adjacent tissues and the presence of distant metastases. Marked nuclear pleomorphism and a high mitotic index are usually but not always characteristics of malignancy; consequently, pathologists must be aware of potential diagnostic pitfalls when assessing the histopathological appearances of tumours. For example, benign tumours arising within endocrine glands often show moderate nuclear pleomorphism while a benign pilomatrixoma of the skin

(a tumour showing differentiation towards skin adnexal structures) characteristically possesses a high mitotic index. By comparison, early cancer of the thyroid gland (follicular carcinoma) shows subtle invasion of adjacent tissues while the tumour cells themselves show minimal nuclear pleomorphism and a low mitotic index.

Tumour stage versus tumour grade

These terms are only used for *malignant* tumours. The grade of a tumour is a measure of the likely aggressiveness of the primary lesion and is only assessable during histological examination of the tumour by a pathologist. The **grade** of a tumour depends upon several linked histopathological features:

- tumour size
- extent of tumour involvement within tissue/organ of origin (e.g. bowel wall)
- tumour involvement of adjacent tissues (e.g. skin)
- metastases within regional or distant lymph nodes
- the number and site of involved lymph nodes may also be important for staging
- presence of metastases within distant tissues other than lymph nodes.

The **stage** of a tumour is an indication of how advanced the growth of the tumour is and may depend on histopathological characteristics of the primary tumour as well as the presence of regional or distant metastases. **Metastases** may be detectable by clinical examination (e.g. palpable enlarged lymph nodes) or additional techniques (e.g. radiological investigations) but confirmation of clinical or radiological abnormalities may require histopathological examination of tissue samples from putative sites of metastasis. Alternatively, histopathological examination of tissues from these sites may reveal microscopic evidence of metastatic disease that was not detectable using clinical or radiological examinations.

Histopathologists, therefore, use tumour features such as growth pattern (differentiation), nuclear pleomorphism and mitotic index both to determine whether tumours are benign or malignant and to assess the grade of malignant tumours (Fig. 3.20.1 and Table 3.20.1). While the range of these features varies among malignant tumours of differing grade, even low-grade (well-differentiated) malignant tumours will generally show a less well-differentiated growth pattern, greater nuclear pleomorphism and a higher mitotic index than 'corresponding' benign tumours.

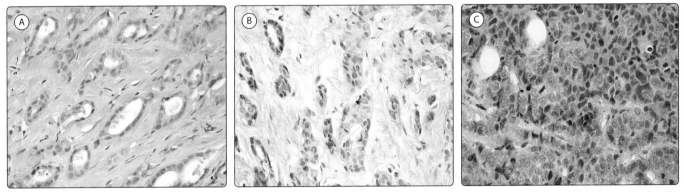

Fig. 3.20.1 Illustrations of breast carcinoma biopsy material to show different grades of invasive carcinoma. (A) Well-differentiated (grade 1) carcinoma cells are forming tubular structures that resemble normal breast ducts, the nuclei show relatively little pleomorphism (variation in size and shape) and no mitotic figures are visible in this section. (B) Moderately differentiated (grade 2) carcinoma cells form some tubules but also exist as cords and islands of cells and there is a greater degree of nuclear pleomorphism. (C) A poorly differentiated (grade 3) the carcinoma; the cells are growing in solid sheets, there is marked nuclear pleomorphism and mitotic figures are visible. Haematoxylin & eosin stain. Magnification ×400.

Table 3.20.1 HISTOPATHOLOGICAL FEATURES COMMONLY IMPORTANT WHEN GRADING MALIGNANT TUMOURS

Tumour cell characteristics	Tumour grade	
	Low grade	High grade
Differentiation	'Well differentiated'	'Poorly differentiated'
Overall growth pattern	Similar to non-neoplastic tissue	Little similarity to non-neoplastic tissue
Nuclear pleomorphism	Mild	Marked
Mitotic index	Low	High

21. Aetiology and epidemiology of neoplasia

Questions
- What causes neoplasms to occur?
- Why don't all neoplasms occur with the same frequency in all populations?
- How can we use our knowledge of the epidemiology of neoplasia to organize healthcare?

Many things contribute to the development of neoplasia, producing a combination of factors that may or may not be under individuals' control (Table 3.21.1). The common theme among these factors is that they result in the accumulation of genetic mutations (see Ch. 22) and defects in the control of cellular proliferation.

Aetiological factors

Genetic abnormalities are very commonly identifiable within neoplastic cells but many of these have occurred after the initiation of neoplasia, within stem cells that possessed a normal genetic constitution and without further cases of the same neoplasm occurring within the same family. However, many neoplasms occur at increased frequency within particular families. In a minority of cases, neoplasia occurs within a family owing to an inherited mutation within a single gene (see also Table 3.22.1):

- *APC* (adenomatous polyposis coli) in familial adenomatous polyposis and colorectal cancer
- *hMLH-1*, *hMSH-2* in hereditary non-polyposis colorectal cancer
- *RB1* in retinoblastoma
- *p53* in Li-Fraumeni syndrome (characterized by the development of multiple malignant tumours, especially sarcomas)
- *BRCA-1* and *BRCA-2* in breast cancer
- *MEN-1* and *MEN-2* in multiple endocrine organ neoplasms.

However, the majority of neoplasms occurring more commonly within affected families arises without a familial pattern suggestive of an inherited defect within a *single* gene. The genetic basis for this observation is not fully understood but it is likely that a combination of mutations within several 'low penetrance' genes accounts for this increased cancer incidence. Colorectal cancer is a good example of familial clustering, with around 25% of cases occurring in families with more than one further case but without evidence of conditions such as familial adenomatous polyposis or hereditary non-polyposis colorectal cancer.

Chemicals can induce neoplasia though the induction of genetic mutations within previously normal cells, for example

- asbestos and malignant mesothelioma
- rubber industry dyes and bladder carcinoma
- cigarette smoke components and lung carcinoma.

The classical model of chemical carcinogenesis proposes phases of neoplasm 'induction' and 'promotion' owing to repeated/long-term exposure to carcinogenic chemicals (Fig. 3.21.1).

Infectious agents can be a potent factor in the development of neoplasia, for example

- human papillomavirus and squamous cell papilloma or cervical carcinoma
- Epstein–Barr virus and malignant lymphoma or nasopharyngeal carcinoma
- liver fluke and cholangiocarcinoma
- *Helicobacter pylori* and gastric lymphoma or gastric carcinoma
- hepatitis B or C viruses and hepatocellular carcinoma
- human herpesvirus 8 and Kaposi's sarcoma.

The mechanism of neoplasia induction varies but a common feature is integration of the genome of the microorganism (especially viral) into that of the host. Infectious agents may also predispose to neoplasia through the development of chronic inflammation and tissue metaplasia. An example is

Table 3.21.1 AETIOLOGICAL FACTORS IN NEOPLASIA DEVELOPMENT

Factor	Clinical example	Neoplasm
Inherited genetic defects	Familial adenomatous polyposis	Colorectal cancer
Exposure to chemical carcinogens	Cigarette smoking	Lung cancer
Infection with certain microorganisms	Human papillomavirus	Cervical cancer
Exposure to forms of radiation	Chernobyl victims	Thyroid cancer

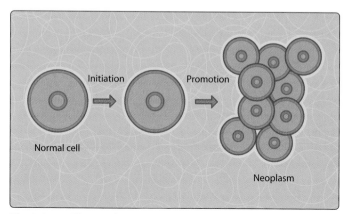

Fig. 3.21.1 Chemical carcinogenesis with phases of induction and promotion owing to repeated/long-term exposure.

schistosomiasis of the bladder, which, when chronic, may induce squamous metaplasia and invasive squamous cell carcinoma within the bladder.

Various forms of **radiation** may induce neoplasia, including ultraviolet radiation, X-rays and emissions from radioactive isotopes (i.e. alpha and beta particles and gamma rays). Patients receive small doses of radiation during investigations such as radiography, computed tomographic (CT) scans and nuclear isotope scans, but the total doses received during these medical tests would not usually significantly increase the risk of neoplasia development. Much larger doses of radiation are received during radiotherapy for cancer and this can increase the risk of developing a second neoplasm. For example, malignant mesothelioma of the pleura or abdomen most commonly occurs in association with asbestos exposure but can exceptionally occur after radiotherapy. Radioactive isotopes may become concentrated within particular organs. For example, children exposed to radiation after the nuclear power station explosion in Chernobyl developed thyroid carcinoma owing to concentration of radioactive iodine within the thyroid gland.

Epidemiology of neoplasia

Much of the epidemiology of neoplasia is explained by differential exposure to aetiological factors. The major factors affecting the incidence of neoplasia are listed in Table 3.21.2. One problems is the time lag between exposure and tumour development. Consequently, while asbestos exposure is now strictly regulated in developed countries, new cases of malignant mesothelioma are still not uncommonly encountered today because of the long time lag (often decades) between asbestos exposure and tumour development.

Environmental factors include the local climate; for example, cutaneous malignant melanoma is particularly common in Australasia where the sunny climate increase the potential exposure to ultraviolet. Colorectal carcinoma is more common in Western populations owing to the low-residue diet, which prolongs bowel transit times and the exposure time to carcinogens within the bowel lumen. Hepatocellular carcinoma is more common in regions such as Southeast Asia where hepatitis B virus infection is widespread. Most neoplasms occur more commonly in older people; this presumably reflects the increased likelihood of significant genetic mutations occurring with increasing age as a result of long-term exposure to risk factors. However, a different well-recognized range of often-aggressive neoplasms arises in childhood, with many occurring only within this age group. Neoplasms of the reproductive system are by definition almost always gender related although 1% of breast carcinomas arise within males.

Gender may be also be related to social factors such as occupation, smoking and alcohol consumption and, therefore, secondarily affect neoplasm incidence. For example, cigarette smoking has until recently been more common among males and this is reflected in the greater incidence of lung carcinoma among men, although an increase in smoking in females has reversed this trend to a degree. Sometimes the living circumstances of an individual result in exposure to multiple risk factors for neoplasia. For example, low social class is associated with poor diet and an increased likelihood of cigarette smoking and excess alcohol consumption.

Using epidemiology to plan healthcare

Our knowledge of the differences in rates of neoplasm incidence between individuals and across populations is important when planning healthcare. For example, advertising campaigns can warn individuals of health risks (e.g. cigarette smoking) or the advantages of being vigilant for early signs of a disease (e.g. breast self-examination). Screening programmes can be devised to enable the early detection of diseases that are common within a population, as long as the characteristics of the diseases are suitable for inclusion within a screening programme (Ch. 30). Highly specific screening programmes can be offered to individuals at known very high risk of certain diseases (e.g. patients with familial adenomatous polyposis have a known extreme risk of developing colorectal cancer; Ch 28). Valuable and often limited resources can be focused on developing and providing the most effective treatments for diseases that are particularly common within a population (e.g. colorectal cancer in Western populations or gastric cancer in Japan).

Table 3.21.2 MAJOR EPIDEMIOLOGICAL FACTORS IN NEOPLASIA

Epidemiological factor	Example
Climate	Cutaneous malignant melanoma
Diet	Colorectal carcinoma
Infections	Hepatocellular carcinoma
Age[a]	Increased incidence in older people; specific childhood tumours
Gender	Reproductive system neoplasms
Cigarette smoking	Lung carcinoma
Excess alcohol consumption	Oral carcinoma
Occupation[b]	Malignant mesothelioma

[a]Most neoplasms occur more commonly in older individuals but specific childhood neoplasms occur almost exclusively early in life.
[b]Strict measures are now imposed to prevent asbestos exposure.

22. Molecular biology of neoplasia

Questions
- What genetic changes occur during the development of neoplasia?
- How can knowledge of genetic changes enhance clinical care?

The development of neoplasms is associated with the gradual accumulation of genetic mutations within the neoplastic cells. Some mutations have no discernable effect while others can lead to serious neoplastic or non-neoplastic diseases. Changes to the genetic material may be substitution or loss of a single DNA nucleotide, a small series of nucleotides or part or the whole of a chromosome (Fig. 3.22.1). Even a single nucleotide substitution can result in gross damage (Fig. 3.22.2). Sometimes a germline (i.e. inherited) genetic mutation is already present within the non-neoplastic cells and this can accelerate the process of neoplastic transformation (Ch. 33). Study of the mutations occurring within neoplastic cell populations can provide an insight into neoplastic transformation and the development into malignancy. Mutations important in the initiation and progression of neoplasia tend to occur within genes whose products are involved in the regulation of cellular growth and differentiation (i.e. the process of maturation from primitive but multipotential stem cells to fully functional and specialized cells).

Genetic mutations and neoplasia

Cells within neoplasms usually contain mutations within multiple genes, most commonly tumour suppressor genes or onco-genes. Mutations spontaneously occur within DNA at a low but significant rate, for example owing to imperfect DNA replication during preparation for cell division. DNA may also accumulate mutations at a higher rate (e.g. in the presence of ionizing radiation). However, many mutations are recognized and corrected by complex intracellular processes, thereby limiting their potentially harmful effects.

Tumour suppressor gene describes a gene whose *normal* function is essential for the prevention of neoplasia development (Table 3.22.1). Although each normal cell contains two copies of each of these genes, only *one* correctly functioning gene is required to prevent neoplasia development. Certain inherited cancer syndromes are characterized by the inheritance of one non-functioning copy of a particular tumour suppressor gene, with mutation of the second copy occurring at the site of tumour development. Knudson was the first to describe this process as the 'two-hit hypothesis', initially in the context of retinoblastoma (a malignant tumour of the retina). Patients with a family history of retinoblastoma (and therefore inheriting a mutation within one copy of the retinoblastoma tumour suppressor gene) developed tumours at a younger age, and more commonly bilaterally, than those without an apparent inherited predisposition. This observation was consistent with the hypothesis that inheritance of one mutated gene was associated with a greater risk of neoplasia since prevention of neoplasia was dependent upon the correct functioning of a single copy of the gene.

Genes whose *normal* function is involved with the control of cellular growth or proliferation are known as **proto-oncogenes**.

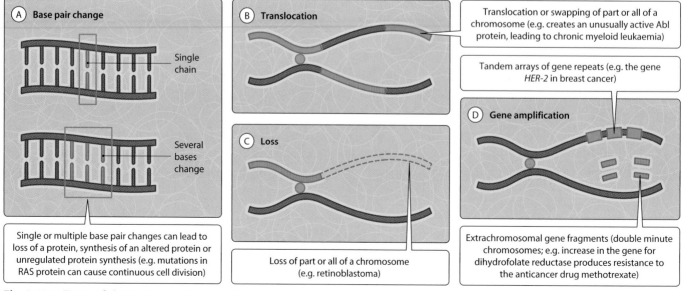

Fig. 3.22.1 Types of change to genetic material.

Mutations that result in the abnormal or uncontrolled activation of proto-oncogenes may lead to neoplasia and in this situation these genes are termed **oncogenes**. Oncogenes contribute to the development of neoplasia through failure of the normal mechanisms regulating cellular growth and proliferation (Table 3.22.2).

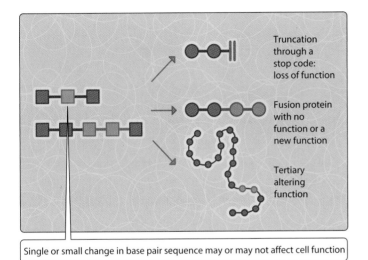

Single or small change in base pair sequence may or may not affect cell function

Truncation through a stop code: loss of function

Fusion protein with no function or a new function

Tertiary altering function

Fig. 3.22.2 Consequences of mutations.

The adenoma–carcinoma sequence

The molecular pathway along which colorectal carcinoma most commonly arises represents an excellent model of the stepwise molecular progression from normal tissue to malignancy. Definition of this pathway has been possible because colorectal carcinoma is known to arise within precursor lesions (adenomas) that are easily identifiable and available for scientific study (Ch. 28). During the progression from normal colonic mucosa to abnormally proliferating (hyperproliferative) mucosa, to adenomas of increasing degrees of dysplasia to invasive carcinoma, a stepwise accumulation of genetic mutations occurs such that early lesions are found to contain one or a small number of mutations and invasive carcinoma contains multiple mutations. The presence of one inherited abnormal copy of a tumour suppressor gene (e.g. a gene encoding a DNA mismatch repair enzyme or the adenomatous polyposis coli (*APC*) gene) increases the likelihood of neoplasia development since the risk of loss of *both* copies is increased. For this reason, patients with inherited cancer syndromes such as hereditary non-polyposis colorectal cancer more commonly develop multiple colorectal carcinomas, or cancer at a younger age, than patients with sporadic cancers.

Table 3.22.1 TUMOUR SUPPRESSOR GENES

Gene	Function	Clinical manifestation[a]
p53	Prevention of cells containing genetic mutations from progressing to mitosis; promotion of apoptosis of these affected cells	Li-Fraumeni syndrome (multiple cancers, especially carcinomas and sarcomas)
hMLH-1, hMSH-2	Repair of genetic mutations	Hereditary non-polyposis colorectal cancer syndrome (especially of proximal colon; endometrial cancer)
RB1	Regulation of the cell cycle	Retinoblastoma, osteosarcoma
APC	Uncertain	Familial adenomatous polyposis
BRCA-1	Growth control	Breast and ovarian cancer
BRCA-2	Uncertain	Breast cancer

[a]Associated with inheritance of germline mutation; however, somatic mutations within some of these genes may also be found in tumour tissue in sporadically occurring cancers.

Table 3.22.2 ONCOGENES

Gene	Mutation	Function	Tumour
bcr–abl	Translocation (9; 22)[a]	Tyrosine kinase activity	Chronic myeloid leukaemia
c-myc	Translocation (8; 14)[b]	Triggers entry into cell cycle	Burkitt's lymphoma
c-erb-B2	Amplification	Growth factor receptor	Breast carcinoma
N-myc	Amplification	Triggers entry into cell cycle	Neuroblastoma
ras	Point mutation[c]	Membrane-bound signal transduction	Colorectal cancer, pancreatic cancer

[a]Formation of the Philadelphia chromosome and a hybrid gene possessing marked tyrosine kinase activity.
[b]The c-myc gene becomes close to the immunoglobulin heavy chain gene (an area with marked transcriptional activity), resulting in abnormally high transcription of c-myc.
[c]Point mutations within the ras family are found in 30% of human cancers.

23. Tumour growth and spread

Questions
- How do tumours grow?
- How does our knowledge of tumour development influence clinical care?

Tumours form through neoplastic transformation of a primitive stem cell within the site of tumour origin. Tumours develop because the growth of these transformed cells has escaped the control mechanisms present within normal cells.

Benign and malignant tumours

Benign tumours grow by forming an expansile mass that gradually compresses adjacent tissues (Fig. 3.23.1 and Table 3.23.1). Examination of benign tumours with the naked eye shows that they are well-circumscribed lesions while histological examination may also reveal a compressed rim of non-neoplastic tissue. Sometimes a rim of fibrous tissue is present at the edge of benign tumours, and this is referred to as a tumour capsule. The clinical effect of compression of adjacent tissues by the tumour depends on the site (Ch. 24). Benign tumours do *not* possess the ability to metastasize to distant sites but they can still cause substantial damage (Table 3.23.2).

Malignant tumours form a mass at their primary site, which may compress but which also characteristically invades into adjacent tissues. The term cancer means crab and was coined in reference to the ability of malignant tumours to infiltrate adjacent tissues with a growth pattern that resembles a crab with long legs and pincers. Malignant tumours often create significant clinical problems at their primary site (Ch. 24) but may additionally spread (**metastasize**) to distant sites. This latter characteristic accounts for most of the mortality associated with malignant tumours and is the subject of much research. Metastasis may occur through one or more of several routes (Table 3.23.3). In order to metastasize, tumour cells must be able to perform certain tasks at different times (Chs 26–29):

1. Detachment of tumour cell from main tumour mass
2. Invasion of detached cell(s) into a vascular or lymphatic space
3. Travel within lymphatic or blood flows to distant site
4. Invasion of vascular/lymphatic space wall and adjacent tissue
5. Tumour cell division and growth of distant metastasis
6. Evasion of host immune response (a key event during the development of all tumours at primary and secondary sites).

Tumour development

Host immunity

In order for tumours to develop, cells must undergo neoplastic transformation while evading attack from the host immune system. **Immunosurveillance** occurs in the normal individual and refers to the process by which certain abnormal proliferations of cells are recognized as such by the immune system and then killed before they can develop into a tumour. Failure of this mechanism is a critical step in tumour development and can occur for several reasons:

- absence of HLA class I molecules on the tumour cell surface
- stimulation of an 'active' T-lymphocyte suppressor mechanism
- induction of 'generalized' immunosuppression
- cytokine-mediated localized immunosuppression.

Failure of immunosurveillance leads to tumour cell growth that is unchecked by the host immune system.

Histological examination of tumours reveals a variable associated inflammatory cell reaction, most commonly comprising lymphocytes and macrophages and present either adjacent to, or directly infiltrating, the tumour. The latter pattern is particularly common in certain tumour types (e.g. malignant melanoma) and results in close approximation of immune cells to tumour cells. Malignant melanomas showing this pattern of inflammatory cell infiltration may also show areas of regression, where partial or even total loss of the tumour mass occurs, presumably as a result of tumour cell killing by the immune cells. Much research is currently focused on the possibility that induction or augmentation of a host response to a tumour may lead to

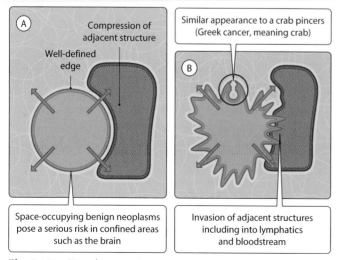

Fig. 3.23.1 Neoplasms. (A) Benign; (B) malignant.

tumour mass reduction and, therefore, represent a new form of cancer treatment (immunotherapy).

Blood supply

Solid tumours, whether benign or malignant, need to retain a sufficiently good blood supply to enable their continued survival and growth. Tumours that outgrow their blood supply cannot survive fully and undergo partial or complete necrosis. The induction and maintenance of a good blood supply is, therefore, critical, and many tumours produce cytokines themselves (e.g. vascular endothelial growth factor) that stimulate the growth of new blood vessels within or immediately adjacent to the tumour (**angiogenesis**). Research is now focused on the possibility of arresting tumour growth by blocking the development of new blood vessels. For example, large benign blood vessel tumours of the skin (haemangiomas) can reduce markedly in size with cytokine treatment (e.g. IL-8) that inhibits angiogenesis.

Table 3.23.1 THE MAJOR DISTINGUISHING FEATURES OF BENIGN AND MALIGNANT TUMOURS

Feature	Benign	Malignant
Cardinal features[a]		
Effect of primary tumour on adjacent tissues	Compression	Invasion
Edge of tumour	Well defined	Poorly defined
Distant metastases	Absent	Present
Other primary features		
Vascular invasion: within lymphatics or blood vessels	Absent	Present
Cellularity: tumour cells per unit area of tumour	Low	High
Nucleus-cytoplasm ratio of tumour cell	Low	High
Differentiation: how much tumour overall growth pattern resembles that of its non-neoplastic counterpart	Good	Variable; often poor
Nuclear pleomorphism: size and shape of nuclei	Mild	Variable; may be marked
Mitotic index: morphological evidence of active cell division	Low	Variable; may be high

[a]Most commonly used to determine biological behaviour of tumours.
[b]Marked nuclear pleomorphism is often associated with an irregular nuclear chromatin pattern and/or nuclear hyperchromasia (dark nuclei as seen on routine H&E staining).

Table 3.23.2 CLINICAL PROBLEMS ARISING ON ADJACENT STRUCTURES

Primary site	Adjacent structure	Clinical problem
Breast	Skin	Ulceration
	Chest wall	Tumour fixation
Brainstem	Cardiovascular centre	Death
Colon	Bladder	Fistula formation
Pancreas	Common bile duct	Obstructive jaundice
Lung	Oesophagus	Dysphagia
	Pulmonary artery	Fatal haemoptysis
Prostate	Prostatic urethra	Urinary retention

Table 3.23.3 ROUTES OF TUMOUR METASTASIS

Route	Sites of metastasis	Clinical example
Lymphatic channels	Local and distant lymph nodes	Axillary node metastases in breast cancer
Blood vessels	Lungs, liver, brain and bone	Cerebral metastasis in lung cancer; bone metastasis in prostatic cancer
Across body cavity	Peritoneum	Carcinomatosis peritonei (widespread foci of metastatic cancer studded across the peritoneal cavity) in colorectal cancer

24. Clinical effects and management of neoplasia

Questions
- What clinical problems do neoplasms create?
- What are the principles of treatment of neoplasms?

Clinical effects

Benign neoplasms

Benign neoplasms usually present because of the local effects of the tumour, with any systemic symptoms linked to the production of a specific chemical such as a hormone by the tumour cells (Table 3.24.1). The clinical effects of benign neoplasms are very dependent upon the site and size of the tumour. Small benign neoplasms are often asymptomatic and only discovered incidentally. However, those occurring at critical sites may cause serious disease or death. Hormone-producing benign tumours most commonly arise within endocrine organs and usually present due to the clinical effects of excess hormone production.

Malignant neoplasms

Malignant neoplasms (cancers) may cause clinical effects from the local primary tumour, from metastases and from the *general* systemic effects of advanced malignancy. Consequently, the clinical sequelae of neoplasms vary, with many causing clinical effects mainly at their primary site but with some more commonly presenting with advanced and widespread disease.

Malignant neoplasms may present with similar **local effects** to those of benign neoplasms. However, malignant neoplasms also possess the ability to invade rather than compress local tissues and this commonly results in their local effects becoming more serious than a benign tumour of the same size occurring at the same site. Malignant neoplasms may, therefore, cause extensive disease locally as well as at a distance through spreading. Figure 3.24.1 shows examples of the problems that can occur depending on the area affected. Adherence, fistula formation, strictures and perforations can all occur in addition to compression.

Metastases may be asymptomatic or may represent the presenting feature of the neoplasm. For example, extensive hepatic metastases may result in few symptoms until the majority of the liver is replaced by tumour. Conversely, a cerebral metastasis may present with neurological problems such as new-onset epilepsy without prior symptoms from the primary tumour. Similarly, a patient may present with a groin mass owing to a lymph node metastasis from a cutaneous malignant melanoma on the leg that had not previously been identified.

The **general symptoms** of advanced malignancy comprise malaise, anorexia and weight loss. The mechanisms behind the development of these symptoms are not fully understood but increased circulating levels of TNF-α is believed to be an important factor. Neoplasms involving the gastrointestinal tract may, of course, contribute more directly to anorexia and weight loss (e.g. via the induction of dysphagia in oesophageal carcinoma).

Management

The treatment of neoplastic disease forms a significant component of modern healthcare. Some neoplasms are treatable using only one form of therapy while others require multiple therapeutic modalities, which may or may not be used sequentially.

Benign neoplasms

Benign neoplasms are potentially curable with complete surgical removal (excision). This is technically possible in many cases (e.g. a fibroadenoma within the breast) while others may be difficult or impossible to remove in their entirety (e.g. a meningioma encroaching upon the brainstem). Some benign neoplasms that are incompletely removed may regrow at their site of origin (local recurrence), although in many cases this does not result in a major clinical problem if the regrowing lesion can once more be surgically removed. The precise site of the neoplasm and the overall fitness of the patient for surgery will help to determine whether the neoplasm can be surgically removed in individual patients. For example, a patient with severe cardiac disease may be unfit for surgical removal of a benign breast neoplasm.

Table 3.24.1 CLINICAL PRESENTATION OF BENIGN NEOPLASMS

Tumour feature	Example	Clinical symptom
Asymptomatic	Renal oncocytoma	Asymptomatic
Pressure on local structures	Pituitary adenoma Osteoma	Tunnel vision Pain
Obstruction of lumen	Ampullary adenoma	Obstructive jaundice
Haemorrhage	Colorectal adenoma Hepatic adenoma	Rectal bleeding Severe intra-abdominal haemorrhage
Hormone production	Pituitary adenoma Adrenocortical adenoma	Acromegaly Cushing's disease, Cushing's syndrome
Malignant transformation	Colorectal adenoma	Colorectal carcinoma

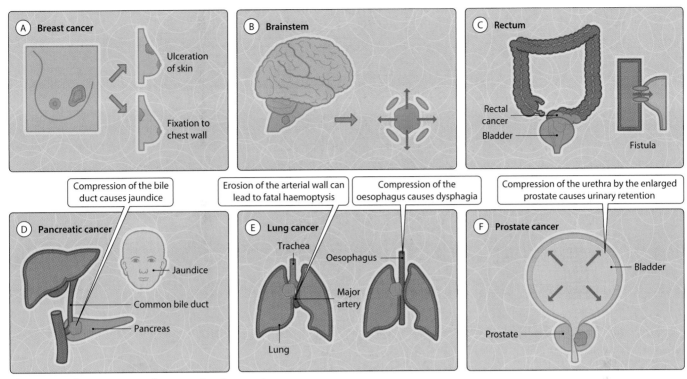

Fig. 3.24.1 Consequences of tumour development.

Malignant neoplasms

Successful treatment of malignant neoplasms requires therapy aimed at the primary lesion and metastatic tumour deposits if present or methods of minimizing the risk of metastasis development if these are not apparent at the time that the primary tumour is undergoing treatment. Like benign neoplasms, the majority of primary malignant neoplasms are best treated using surgical excision. Invasion of adjacent tissues may make surgical removal difficult or impossible.

Surgical excision is the most common treatment of choice for removal of the primary malignant tumour, locally invaded adjacent structures and regional lymph node metastases. Isolated distant metastases (e.g. within the brain, lung and liver) are often not curable but may also be amenable to surgical removal. **Radiotherapy** can be used to treat primary tumours that are not surgically removable (e.g. deep within the brain) or after surgery to reduce the risk of local tumour recurrence (e.g. after local removal of breast cancer). Radiotherapy can also be used prior to surgery to reduce the size of an otherwise inoperable primary tumour, making it more amenable to surgical excision. **Chemotherapy** is the treatment of choice for leukaemias and most lymphomas. Chemotherapy may also be used alone or in combination with radiotherapy prior to surgery, or after surgery in patients at high risk of distant tumour metastasis.

All modalities of cancer treatment are continually advancing and additional methods include hormonal therapy (e.g. medical anti-oestrogen therapy for breast cancer) and novel medical treatments that interrupt vital pathways of tumour cell growth induction (e.g. inhibitors of tyrosine kinase growth factor receptors for leukaemia or gastrointestinal stromal tumours; blocking agents for the HER-2 growth factor receptor for breast cancer).

The initial aim of most cancer treatments is to provide the highest chance of a complete cure. However, some patients present with already advanced malignancy with widespread local and/or metastatic disease. In these patients, as well as those whose disease has advanced despite potentially curative treatment, many therapeutic options are available to slow the further progress of the neoplasm and/or to alleviate distressing symptoms, even if cure is no longer possible. Surgery may be used to reduce tumour bulk (e.g. brain tumours that cause pressure on adjacent structures) or to bypass segments of the gastrointestinal tract that are blocked by a neoplasm. Radiotherapy and chemotherapy may be used to reduce the size of inoperable primary tumours or to shrink metastases: radiotherapy may be particularly effective in reducing pain caused by skeletal metastases. Important medical treatments include adequate pain relief and anti-emetic (anti-nausea) agents as well as specific treatment of distressing symptoms such as excessive saliva production. The treatment of patients with incurable neoplastic (or non-neoplastic) disease is termed **palliative care** and represents a medical speciality in its own right. Palliative care doctors and nurses are very important members of extended multidisciplinary cancer teams and work within both hospital and community settings.

25. Prognostic factors in neoplasia

Questions
- How do neoplasms cause death?
- How do we predict the clinical behaviour of neoplasms?

The predicted clinical outcome for a patient with a particular disease is referred to as their **prognosis** and depends on the nature of the disease process and the general medical condition of the patient. The prognosis of all diseases is based upon our understanding of their pathophysiology and our experience of clinical outcomes in previous patients. A prognosis can be expressed in several ways, such as the likelihood of disease recurrence or progression, the average period of disease-free survival or the overall likelihood of survival for a certain time period.

The accuracy with which a prognosis can be calculated varies considerably between diseases. Medical interventions (i.e. treatments) may be considered successful if they improve the patient's prognosis, although some treatments are designed to be purely supportive in nature, ameliorating distressing symptoms such as severe pain but not necessarily altering the course of the disease. The latter may apply to patients with incurable conditions, which may be neoplastic (e.g. widespread cancer) or non-neoplastic (e.g. motor neuron disease) in nature.

Neoplasia and mortality

Malignant tumours most commonly cause death through the development of metastases within vital organs such as the brain and liver. Therefore, although the primary tumour may result in distressing symptoms, treatment of malignant tumours always aims to reduce the risk of metastasis occurring or to reduce the size of established metastases. Malignant tumours may also cause death through extensive local growth and infiltration of adjacent tissues. Oesophageal carcinomas often cause dysphagia (difficulty swallowing) by obstructing the oesophageal lumen, and this contributes to the severe weight loss characteristic of this disease. Colonic carcinomas may cause bowel obstruction or perforation, with peritonitis. Lung cancers not uncommonly grow into the walls of major mediastinal blood vessels such as the aorta with massive ensuing haemoptysis (coughing up blood). Cerebral gliomas almost never metastasize beyond the central nervous system (although they may widely disseminate within the brain and spinal cord) but result in damage to the cardiovascular and respiratory centres within the brainstem, either by direct infiltration or through secondary effects of raised intracranial pressure.

Benign tumours cannot metastasize but may still unusually cause death by compression of vital adjacent structures. Even a small benign tumour within or next to the brainstem (e.g. a meningioma) may lead to death through damage to the cardiovascular or respiratory centres.

Factors affecting prognosis

The prognosis of a neoplastic disease is dependent upon characteristics of the tumour and the 'host' (the patient) (Table 3.25.1). **Pathological factors** in prognosis include:
- primary tumour position
- primary tumour type
- primary tumour size
- primary tumour grade (applicable only to malignant tumours)
- tumour stage, including extent of primory tumour.

Clinical factors affecting prognosis include
- patient age
- additional disease processes (e.g. serious underlying diseases such as ischaemic heart disease or chronic lung disease).

The presence of additional non-neoplastic diseases (**comorbidity**) may adversely affect prognosis both directly and indirectly. For example, the presence of coexistent serious lung disease may entirely preclude a major surgical procedure to remove an otherwise 'operable' neoplasm such as localized colorectal cancer, or it may significantly increase the risk of death following such surgery. This means that patients with significant comorbidity may be offered a different treatment, such as radiotherapy, which may be associated with a lower chance of 'cure' than major surgery. It should also be borne in mind that the best treatment for some tumours is a non-surgical method and in appropriate circumstances these may be associated with excellent survival (e.g. invasive squamous cell carcinoma of the anal canal, which can respond dramatically to radiotherapy alone or in combination with chemotherapy).

Examples of prognosis determination

Most benign tumours (apart from the exceptions described above) are associated with an excellent prognosis, with successful removal almost always resulting in a complete 'cure'. The prognosis of malignant tumours is extremely variable between tumours. Some malignant neoplasms are almost universally associated with a very poor prognosis. Examples include small cell carcinoma of the lung, glioblastoma multiforme of the brain or adenocarcinoma of the pancreas. Although modern treatments can prolong the survival of patients with aggressive neoplasms of poor prognosis, the 5-year survival rate for tumours such as these is generally 0–15%. However, many malignant tumours are associated with a much better prognosis, either because of the indolent (slowly progressive) nature of the tumour or because of the development of highly effective modern treatments. Examples of the latter are malignant germ cell neoplasms of the testis, in which combinations of surgery, radiotherapy and chemotherapy now commonly result in 'cures' even when patients present with disseminated (i.e. advanced tumours with metastatic spread) disease. The precise factors determining patient survival are becoming increasingly clear. Prognostication has been particularly well characterized for some common tumours; an example is for surgically excised colorectal cancers where prognosis is directly related to the tumour stage (Ch. 28).

Cancer staging: the TNM system

Stage is one of the most important prognostic factors in malignant neoplasms, and the treatment patients receive often varies according to the stage of the disease. Therefore, classifying malignant neoplasms according to stage is one of the main goals in managing patients with cancer.

The Dukes staging system for colorectal carcinoma is discussed in Ch. 28. Another commonly used system is TNM. There are TNM classifications for most common cancers. Although the details of the TNM classifications for each cancer vary from one site to another, the principle is the same at all sites: the T category shows how far the tumour has spread locally; the N category shows whether there is involvement of regional nodes; and the M category shows whether there is distant metastasis. For example, in the colon, a carcinoma that is classified as T2 N1 M0 is one that has spread into the muscularis propria but not beyond it (T2), has involved between 1 and 3 lymph nodes (N1), but has not produced any distant metastases, e.g. in liver or lung (M0). The TNM categories can then be used to place cancers into stage groups that reflect prognosis and response to treatment.

Table 3.25.1 MAJOR FACTORS AFFECTING PROGNOSIS IN NEOPLASIA

	Good prognostic factors	Poor prognostic factors
Tumour characteristics	Most benign tumour types	Benign tumours in sites where they can compress vital structures
	Malignant tumours	Particularly high grade (histologically aggressive), advanced stage (e.g. large, metastases present), invading blood or lymphatic channel
Host characteristics		
Age[a]	Young	Older
Other disease processes	None	Present, e.g. cardiovascular disease, chronic lung disease
Access to good-quality healthcare	Yes	No

[a]Among adults, patients who are younger are generally more likely to be otherwise relatively fit and less likely to possess serious disease within other organ systems. Paradoxically, some neoplasias (e.g. breast cancer) appear to behave more aggressively when they arise in younger patients; therefore, young age is not always a good prognostic factor. Furthermore, some neoplasms only occur in children and young adults (Ch. 31).

26. Lung cancer

Questions
- Why does lung cancer occur?
- What are its clinical and pathological features?
- How can we treat lung cancer?

Lung cancer is the most common cause of cancer deaths among men in Western populations and may soon overtake breast cancer as the most common cause of cancer deaths among women.

Aetiological factors

Cigarette smoking is overwhelmingly the most common aetiological factor for primary lung cancer, which is exceedingly rare among non-smokers, in whom it is often linked to passive smoking. Primary lung cancer most commonly develops during the sixth to eighth decades but may also occur in younger individuals, especially those who are heavy cigarette smokers. Asbestos exposure is a potent risk factor for lung carcinoma, with cancer in affected patients often developing many years or even decades after asbestos exposure.

Clinical presentation

Primary lung cancer may present clinically with intractable cough, breathlessness or haemoptysis (coughing up blood). However, presentation owing to metastatic disease (e.g. neurological symptoms, jaundice) or the general symptoms of advanced malignancy (e.g. anorexia, severe weight loss) is common. Clinical examination may reveal cachexia or an enlarged liver while a chest X-ray usually reveals the primary tumour as a lung mass. The diagnosis may be confirmed using cytology (e.g. identification of malignant cells within sputum) or histopathology (e.g. needle core biopsy of the lung lesion).

Pathological features

Primary lung cancers are almost always carcinomas, although other tumours such as malignant lymphomas may exceptionally originate within the lung. Lung carcinomas are often macroscopically obvious tumours several centimetres in size, although sometimes primary lung carcinomas a few millimetres across may give rise to widely disseminated malignancy. The most common histological types of lung carcinoma are small cell and non-small cell types, with the latter subdivided into squamous cell carcinoma, adenocarcinoma and undifferentiated carcinoma. Mixtures between all histological types is not uncommonly seen. The tumours may invade local structures, metastasize via lymphatic channels to regional or distant lymph nodes and via the blood to distant sites (Fig. 3.26.1).

Treatment

Lung carcinoma is usually an aggressive form of cancer from which a full recovery is unusual, although not impossible. The primary tumours often directly invade local structures such as the mediastinum and chest wall and commonly metastasize to mediastinal lymph nodes and via the bloodstream to distant organs. Surgery (e.g. partial or complete pneumonectomy) offers the best chance of a cure but many patients present with disseminated disease that is not amenable to surgical excision. Radiotherapy and chemotherapy are usually used as palliative treatments for patients with advanced disease but may sometimes produce an excellent reduction in tumour size, especially in small cell and squamous cell carcinoma.

Primary versus metastatic tumours

The lung is also a common site for the development of metastatic tumour deposits from primary tumours that disseminate via the bloodstream. The number of possible primary sites for a metastatic tumour within the lung is, therefore, very large but the most common sites of origin for such tumours would include carcinomas of the gastrointestinal tract, breast and prostate gland and malignant melanoma. The correct interpretation of a lung tumour as primary or metastatic in nature requires a careful clinical assessment together with a radiological search for distant tumours and detailed histological examination of a tissue sample from the tumour. Assessment using a panel of immunohistochemical markers can nowadays help to determine the putative primary site of metastatic tumours in many cases, and this information can be used to determine prognosis and determine subsequent patient management.

Smoking and lung cancer

The association between cigarette smoking and lung cancer is now very well established, but the way in which this association became understood is an excellent example of the importance of epidemiology. The *British Doctors Study*, initiated in 1951 by Sir Richard Doll and Ashley Hill in Oxford, provided key evidence for the link between smoking and lung cancer. This study followed a cohort of 35 000 male doctors in the UK, providing statistical proof of this disease link initially in 1956 but incredibly continuing to follow the same cohort of doctors until 2001. The final publication of data from this study in 2004 revealed that smoking reduces life expectancy by up to 10 years, not only through lung cancer but also from the development of other smoking-related diseases such as ischaemic heart disease and chronic lung disease.

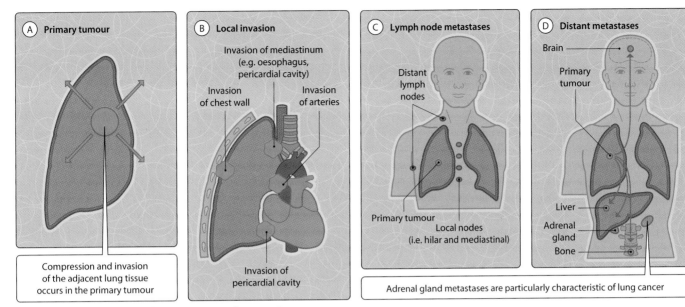

Fig. 3.26.1 The progression of lung cancer from a primary tumour.

LUNG CANCER

A 62-year-old man presented with marked vascular engorgement and swelling of his head, neck and upper limbs. He had smoked 30 cigarettes daily for 40 years. A chest radiograph and subsequent CT scan revealed a 4 cm mass within the right lung that was extending into the mediastinum and compressing the superior vena cava. Metastatic tumour deposits were identified within four ribs. Histopathological examination of a core biopsy of the mass revealed small cell carcinoma of presumed primary origin within the lung. Since this tumour type is known to be sensitive to chemotherapy and radiotherapy, the patient was given emergency radiotherapy, which significantly reduced the size of the main tumour mass and alleviated the obstruction of the superior vena cava. He was subsequently given chemotherapy, which reduced the size of the main tumour mass further and resulted in disappearance of the distant metastases on follow-up CT scan. The tumour subsequently recurred 2 years later and he died with widespread metastases 2.5 years after the initial diagnosis. However, his survival was considerably longer than the few days that he would have survived had he not been treated with radiotherapy and chemotherapy.

27. Breast cancer

Questions
- Why does breast cancer occur?
- What are its clinical and pathological features?
- How can we treat breast cancer?

Breast cancer is the second most common cause of cancer deaths in industrialized societies. The disease most commonly affects women during the fifth to seventh decades but may affect young women and even adolescents.

Aetiological factors

Breast cancer is a common malignancy and, therefore, it is not uncommon to find more than one affected individual within families. However, predisposition to breast cancer is conferred by a specific inherited genetic defect in a small minority (less than 5%). Studies of large family trees led to the discovery of the *BRCA-1* and *BRCA-2* genes, mutations within which have been shown to be associated with a very high risk of breast cancer development. Mutations may occur at many different positions within these genes. Females from families possessing such inherited mutations require especially careful screening for breast cancer. Affected individuals may develop breast cancer at an early age (e.g. the third decade) and the cancers that develop often show characteristic (but not entirely specific) features.

Several other clinicopathological factors apart from an inherited predisposition are associated with an increased risk of breast cancer development. Many of these factors result in increased exposure of breast tissue to circulating oestrogens. Such factors include obesity, early menarche, late menopause and nulliparity. Cancer within one breast is associated with an increased risk of cancer within the contralateral breast, suggesting that a 'field change' has occurred within the patient's breast tissue.

Clinical presentation

Breast cancer mostly presents clinically from the primary tumour, most commonly as a breast mass but sometimes with breast pain or a nipple discharge. The disease may, however, present at an advanced stage with symptoms of the metastases (e.g. epilepsy from a cerebral metastasis; Fig. 3.27.1).

Pathological features

Breast cancer may exist as preinvasive in-situ disease, in which cancer cells are contained within the breast ducts and lobules, or as invasive disease in which the cancer cells have progressed beyond the confines of the ductal and lobular system into the surrounding connective tissue. Invasive breast cancer may grow directly into the overlying skin or the chest wall, metastasize via lymphatics to regional axillary or internal mammary artery lymph nodes or metastasize via the bloodstream to distant organs (Fig. 3.27.1).

The histological growth pattern of in-situ and invasive breast cancers is diverse but 75% of invasive breast cancers are classed as **ductal** in type. Accurate pathological assessment of tumour grade and stage is essential for correct patient management. The grade of a breast cancer is a histological assessment of the aggressiveness of the tumour. The stage of the tumour is an assessment of how advanced the disease process is and is

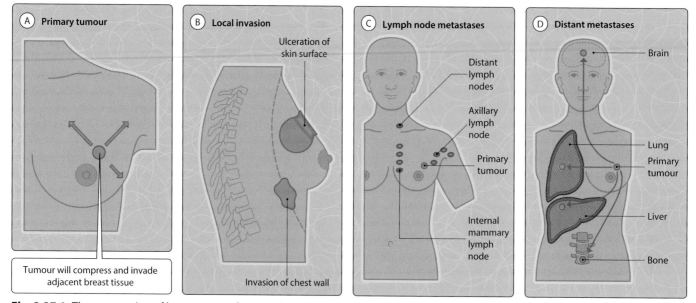

Fig. 3.27.1 The progression of breast cancer from a primary tumour.

dependent upon the characteristics of the primary tumour together with the presence of regional or distant metastases. Prognosis is linked to both the tumour grade and the stage, with high-grade and/or high-stage tumours behaving the most aggressively and associated with a worse clinical outcome. The detailed histological features affecting prognosis in invasive breast carcinoma have been particularly well characterized (Table 3.27.1).

Pathologists can further help to determine prognosis for patients with breast cancer by determining the hormone receptor and growth factor receptor (**HER-2**) status of the tumour, using immunohistochemistry. Approximately 75% of invasive breast carcinomas express **oestrogen receptors** within the nucleus of the carcinoma cells and a similar proportion express progesterone receptors. The growth of tumours expressing these receptors is usually dependent on circulating oestrogens and progression of the tumours can often be slowed significantly using drugs that block the effect of oestrogens on the carcinoma cells (e.g. tamoxifen) or reduce the production of circulating oestrogens (e.g. anastrazole). HER-2 is a growth factor receptor expressed on the cytoplasmic membranes of the carcinoma cells in abnormally high quantities in approximately 30% of invasive breast cancers. Overexpression of this receptor is associated with poor prognosis but also predicts response to the specific growth factor receptor-blocking agent trastuzumab (Herceptin).

Treatment

Pure in-situ breast carcinoma has no propensity to metastasize and is curable by surgical excision. Invasive breast cancer may also be curable by surgical excision, usually combined with radiotherapy to reduce the risk of local tumour recurrence. Long-term patient survival in invasive breast cancer is dependent on the prevention of distant metastases. Therefore, suitable patients in whom regional lymph node metastases are identified on pathological examination are usually offered chemotherapy. The growth of many breast cancers is dependent upon stimulation of the tumour cells by oestrogens. Therefore, anti-oestrogen therapies such as tamoxifen may be very effective in preventing disease progression.

Breast cancer screening

Screening asymptomatic individuals for breast cancer can result in a significant fall in mortality from this disease. The NHS Breast Screening Programme invites women aged 50–70 years for mammography every 3 years. The aim of breast cancer screening is to detect the disease at the in-situ or early invasive stage, when prompt treatment is associated with improved survival. Breast cancer may be detected on mammograms as tiny foci of calcification (**microcalcification**; most commonly seen within ductal carcinoma in situ) or masses/deformities (most commonly seen in invasive breast cancer). Women in whom these abnormalities are detected are recalled for further assessment, which comprises clinical and detailed radiological examinations. Fine needle aspiration cytology or needle core biopsy examination of the abnormal area of tissue is often performed at this time and may lead to surgical removal of the abnormality.

Table 3.27.1 MAJOR HISTOLOGICAL PROGNOSTIC FACTORS IN INVASIVE BREAST CARCINOMA

Tumour characteristic	Good prognosis	Poor prognosis
Tumour type[a]	Tubular carcinoma	Metaplastic carcinoma
Tumour size	Small; especially < 10 mm	Large
Tumour grade	1	3
Vascular invasion by tumour	Absent	Present
Lymph node metastases	No	Yes
Hormone receptor status	Oestrogen receptor positive	Oestrogen receptor negative
Growth factor receptor (HER-2) status	Negative	Positive

[a]Histologically, 75% are classified as invasive ductal carcinoma; certain unusual histological subtypes possess a better or worse prognosis than invasive ductal carcinoma as illustrated here.

BREAST CANCER

A 50-year-old woman presented with a breast mass, and histopathological examination of a core biopsy of the mass revealed an invasive carcinoma. Wide local excision of the mass was performed and histopathological examination revealed a 20 mm grade 3 invasive ductal carcinoma extending to 1 mm from the edge of the specimen (a risk factor for local tumour recurrence). Five of the eighteen lymph nodes identified within an axillary lymph node dissection specimen contained foci of metastatic tumour (a risk factor for distant tumour metastasis). Immunohistochemical staining performed on histological sections of the tumour revealed that it was oestrogen receptor positive. The pathologist communicated these results to the breast surgeon and oncologist at the multidisciplinary team meeting. The patient was given radiotherapy to the breast to reduce the risk of local recurrence and chemotherapy to reduce the risk of distant metastasis. Since the tumour was oestrogen receptor positive she was also treated with anti-oestrogen medical therapy. Despite these treatments, the patient developed bony metastases 3 years later that were unresponsive to further conventional chemotherapy. Additional immunohistochemical staining of histological sections of the tumour revealed that it was HER-2 positive and, therefore, she was started on trastuzumab (Herceptin) therapy, which reduced the size of her bone metastases.

28. Colorectal cancer

Questions
- Why does colorectal cancer occur?
- What are its clinical and pathological features?
- How can we treat colorectal cancer?

The most common cancer of the large intestine is adenocarcinoma. This lesion is more common in Western than non-Western societies and is the third most common cancer in the UK.

Aetiological factors
Genetic and environmental factors contribute to the development of colorectal cancer. Around 25% of cases show 'familial clustering' but less than 5% occur in association with a clearly identifiable genetic mutation (Table 3.28.1). A low-residue 'Western' diet is thought to increase the risk of colorectal cancer by increasing bowel content transit time.

Almost all colorectal carcinomas develop from precursor lesions termed **adenomas**. Colonic adenomas are polypoid or flat lesions in which the epithelium shows variable degrees of dysplasia. The development of adenomas from normal mucosa and their subsequent progression to malignant invasion is termed the adenoma–carcinoma sequence (Chs 22 and 33).

Clinical presentation
As with all malignant tumours, patients with colorectal carcinoma may present with symptoms caused by the primary tumour, the metastases or the general features of malignancy (Fig. 3.28.1). Carcinomas may appear to the naked eye as polyps, malignant ulcers (i.e. with rolled everted edges) or areas of stricture formation (i.e. wall thickening with bowel lumenal narrowing). Typical effects of a primary tumour are change in bowel habit, rectal bleeding and/or mucus, anaemia, abdominal mass, bowel obstruction/perforation and fistula formation. Metastases cause jaundice (colorectal carcinoma is a relatively common cause of liver metastases, which can present before the primary tumour is identified, for example with jaundice), cerebral disturbance (brain metastases) and bone pain (skeletal metastases). In addition, there will be the general features of malignancy: tiredness, weight loss, anorexia and anaemia. Although anaemia can occur through chronic haemorrhage from small and large intestinal tumours or from the general effects of advanced malignancy, it is a particularly common (and often the only) feature of malignancy occurring within the caecum and ascending colon. Bowel perforation or acute obstruction are surgical emergencies in which the patient usually presents acutely unwell and commonly with the clinical features of an 'acute abdomen'.

Pathological features
Although histological examination reveals that the vast majority of colorectal cancers are adenocarcinomas, other types of cancer may be encountered occasionally. Carcinomas spread through the bowel wall, and if they penetrate the peritoneal surface they may then spread across the peritoneal cavity with widespread seeding of tumour (trans-coelomic spread). Metastasis occurs via lymphatic vessels to regional mesenteric lymph nodes and via blood vessels to distant organs (especially the liver but also the brain, lungs and bone; Fig. 3.28.1). The Dukes staging system was first developed for rectal cancer and is now still used in updated form by many surgeons and pathologists for staging colorectal cancer (Table 3.28.2). Accurate tumour staging, now most commonly achieved using the internationally recognized TNM (Ch. 25) system, is essential for prognosis and treatment options. Preoperative tumour staging is performed using radiological investigations (e.g. CT and magnetic resonance imaging (MRI) of the abdomen and pelvis) but the definitive tumour stage can only be calculated after careful pathological examination of the resected bowel specimen.

Table 3.28.1 GENETIC PREDISPOSITION TO COLORECTAL ADENOCARCINOMA

Condition	Inheritance	Prevalence (%)	Gene(s) involved	Clinical
Familial clustering	Not defined	25	Multiple uncharacterized genes	
Familial adenomatous polyposis	Autosomal dominant	< 5	APC (adenomatous polyposis coli)	Multiple colorectal polyps and early colorectal cancer; other carcinomas, e.g. small bowel
Hereditary non-polyposis colorectal cancer syndrome	Autosomal dominant	< 5	DNA mismatch repair enzymes, e.g. hMLH-1, hMSH-2	Age < 50 years; proximal tumours more common; other carcinomas, e.g. endometrial

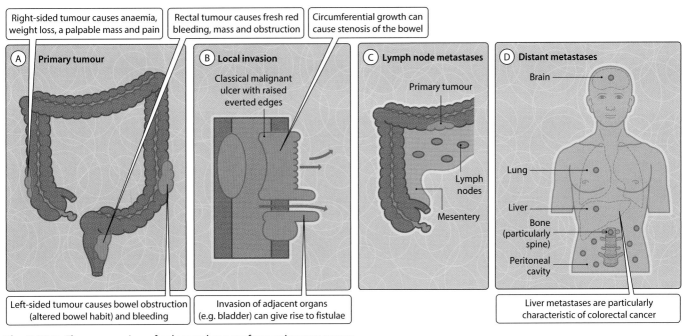

Fig. 3.28.1 The progression of colorectal cancer from primary tumour.

Treatment

Curative treatment usually comprises surgical excision of the involved bowel segment together with radiotherapy or chemotherapy if required. Chemotherapy is usually offered to suitable patients if regional lymph node metastases are identified as this reduces the risk of distant metastases. Radiotherapy may be given preoperatively to patients with bulky rectal cancers in order to increase the chance of subsequent curative surgical excision or it may be used postoperatively if pathological examination of the resection specimen reveals a rectal tumour with an otherwise high risk of local recurrence.

Table 3.28.2 MODIFIED DUKES' STAGING SYSTEM FOR COLORECTAL ADENOCARCINOMA

Dukes' stage	Features	5-year survival (%)
A	Primary tumour does not penetrate the full thickness of muscularis propria; regional lymph nodes negative	90
B	Primary tumour penetrates full thickness of muscularis propria; regional lymph nodes negative	60
C	Regional lymph node metastases present	30
D	Distant (e.g. liver) metastases present	5–10

COLORECTAL CANCER

A 57-year-old man presented with rectal bleeding and changes in bowel habit and investigations (including histopathological examination of a rectal biopsy) revealed adenocarcinoma of the rectum. He underwent anterior resection of the rectum (removal of the rectum via an incision in the anterior abdominal wall). Histopathological examination revealed that the tumour had invaded through the full thickness of the bowel wall and that tumour was present at the circumferential surgical margin (i.e. the edge of the specimen; a risk factor for local tumour recurrence within the pelvis). Tumour foci were also present within 3 of 15 lymph nodes that were found within the resection specimen (a risk factor for distant tumour metastasis). The pathologist communicated these findings to the colorectal surgeon and oncologist at the colorectal cancer multidisciplinary team meeting and, as a result, the patient was given radiotherapy to the pelvis to reduce the risk of local tumour recurrence and chemotherapy to reduce the risk of distant metastases.

29. Prostatic cancer

Questions
- Why does prostatic cancer occur?
- What are its clinical and pathological features?
- How can we treat prostatic cancer?

Prostatic cancer is one of the most common forms of malignancy among males. The incidence has apparently increased in recent years although this may be at least partly reflect increased diagnosis of early cancer within screening programmes. The disease primarily affects men in their sixth to ninth decades but may also occur in younger individuals.

Aetiological factors

The precise aetiology of prostate cancer has not yet been determined. However, increased exposure of prostatic epithelium to circulating oestrogens, as occurs in late middle-aged and elderly men, is believed to be an important factor in cancer development.

Clinical presentation

Prostate cancer may present with bladder outflow obstruction as a result of the prostatic enlargement (Fig. 3.29.1) and may be diagnosed incidentally during histological examination of tissue chippings removed at transurethral surgery for an enlarged prostate gland. Advanced cancer may present with metastatic disease (e.g. bone pain from skeletal metastases). An increasing number of patients are now diagnosed during specific screening for this disease (see below). Clinical examination in prostate cancer may reveal an asymmetrically enlarged firm prostate gland on digital rectal examination. Isotope bone scanning is commonly used to search for bony metastases.

Pathological features

Advanced prostatic cancer results in marked, often asymmetrical, enlargement of the prostate gland while early cancer is only identifiable under histological examination. Almost all prostatic cancers are adenocarcinomas and the tumour grade is determined by the histopathological growth pattern. The tumour may develop as an expansile nodule within the prostate gland or as a diffusely infiltrative mass with extension beyond the glandular capsule and growth into adjacent tissues. Tumour cell invasion of the perineural space surrounding nerves is a particular characteristic of prostatic cancer and is one of the factors resulting in local tumour recurrence after radical surgery. The tumours metastasize via lymphatics to regional lymph nodes (especially pelvic and retroperitoneal nodes) and via the bloodstream to distant sites; skeletal metastases appearing as sclerotic (i.e. dense) lesions on radiological survey or bone scanning are particularly common in advanced disease.

Treatment

Early prostatic cancer, most commonly detected within screening programmes, may be amenable to surgical excision (**radical prostatectomy**: removal of the whole prostate gland via an incision in the anterior abdominal wall, with removal of several pelvic lymph nodes) when radiological examination demonstrates that the tumour is contained within the prostate gland. Patients with more advanced tumours or otherwise unsuitable for surgery may benefit from radiotherapy; this is increasingly delivered nowadays via radioactive wires inserted into the prostate gland (**brachytherapy**). Hormonal manipulation therapy may also be successful either alone or in combination with the above treatments. Monitoring of the serum **prostate serum antigen** (PSA) concentration is a very useful method of monitoring response to treatment: a rise in PSA in these circumstances often means that local disease recurrence or distant metastasis has occurred.

Prostate cancer screening

The advent of prostate cancer screening has very significantly increased the proportion of new cases identified at an early, asymptomatic stage within screened populations. When

PROSTATE CANCER

A 48-year-old man was found to have a raised serum PSA at a health screen. Ultrasound examination revealed a nodular prostate gland with one 10 mm area showing a particularly abnormal ultrasound signal. Ultrasound-guided transrectal core biopsy of the prostate gland was performed and histopathological examination revealed the presence of well-differentiated prostatic adenocarcinoma. A CT scan revealed that the tumour appeared to be contained within the prostate gland and no distant metastases were identified. The patient, therefore, underwent a radical prostatectomy. Histopathological examination of the removed gland revealed that although most of the tumour was contained within the gland, carcinoma extended through the gland capsule in one small area and reached the edge of the specimen. Therefore the patient was given radiotherapy to reduce the risk of local tumour recurrence. However, the 10 lymph nodes examined showed no evidence of tumour involvement and, therefore, the risk of future distant tumour spread was assessed as low and the patient's prognosis as good.

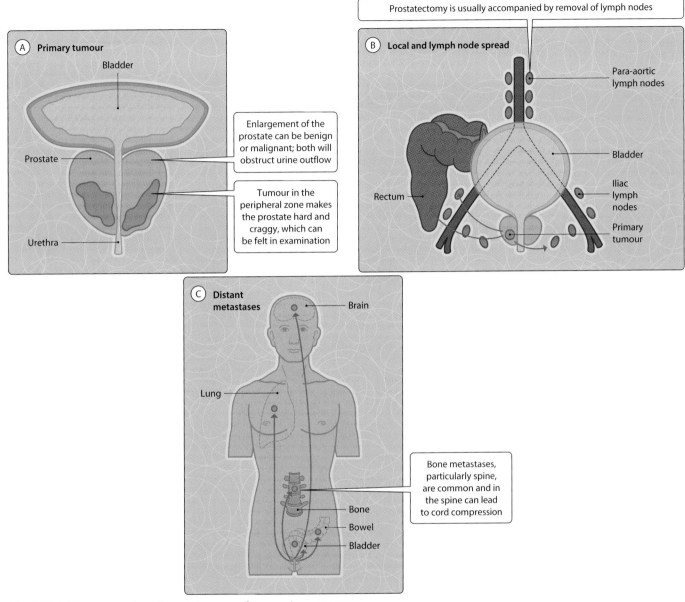

Fig. 3.29.1 The progression of prostate cancer from a primary tumour.

available, screening is currently offered to middle-aged and elderly men and involves regular measurements of serum PSA within peripheral blood samples. This is a sensitive marker of prostatic disease, with modest rises in PSA occurring in prostatitis and more marked elevations usually signifying the onset of malignancy.

Men in whom a raised PSA level is found undergo clinical examination (rectal examination) together with transrectal ultrasound examination of the prostate gland with multiple needle core biopsies of the gland taken for histological examination.

30. Principles of disease screening

Questions
- What does screening mean?
- What criteria does a disease need to fulfil in order to be detected by screening?

Screening for a disease means searching for evidence of that disease among asymptomatic individuals. The aim of screening is to detect a disease at an early stage, when treatment is associated with an improved outcome (i.e. a better chance of survival from the disease) compared with the outcome if a patient presented with symptoms of the disease.

Criteria of suitability for screening

Several criteria have to be fulfilled in order for a disease to be potentially suitable for screening:

- the biological progression must be understood
- an asymptomatic phase must exist
- the screening test must be acceptable to the individual
- the programme must be cost effective
- the screening test must be as sensitive and specific as possible
- detection of the disease at an early stage must be associated with improved survival
- a suitable treatment for the disease should exist, if detected by screening
- the potential impact of the disease on the population needs to be significant.

The requirement for a significant impact on the population means that the disease should be common and/or associated with serious consequences for affected individuals. The biological progression of the disease is important; in particular, a presymptomatic phase must exist during which the early disease process can be identified by a suitable screening test. Tests must have a high degree of:

- **sensitivity** (a **low false-negative rate**): should identify as many affected individuals as possible
- **specificity** (a **low false-positive rate**): should be negative in individuals not affected by the disease.

The test should be acceptable to the individuals to be screened (e.g. not unnecessarily invasive or painful). An effective management strategy must exist for the disease; this will usually comprise treatment although for incurable inherited diseases (e.g. Huntington's disease) it could comprise appropriate counselling. Where treatment is offered to presymptomatic individuals, this should be associated with an improved clinical outcome compared with treatment offered to patients presenting with symptoms from the disease. Finally, the cost of the screening programme should be justifiable in terms of the reduction in mortality or increase in quality of life that is resultant to individuals entering the programme.

Screening programmes

The NHS Cervical Screening Programme

The NHS Cervical Screening Programme was initiated in the 1960s and comprises periodic cervical cytology (i.e. examination of cervical smears). The aim is to detect cervical carcinoma at an early preinvasive stage (i.e. cervical intraepithelial neoplasia), during which time complete excision of the abnormal epithelium is potentially curative. A cervical smear is obtained by gently scraping the cervix with a wooden spatula after visualization of the cervix using a vaginal speculum (Fig. 2.30.1). The mucus scraped from the cervix contains exfoliated cells, which are spread onto microscope slides, stained and visualized under a microscope (Fig. 3.30.2). It is currently planned that a newer technique, termed liquid-based cytology, will be introduced widely across the UK; this is a method of enhancing the quality of cervical cytology specimens by rinsing the harvested cells into a liquid medium and then evenly distributing the cells across a microscope slide.

Cytological examination involves careful assessment of the characteristics of individual cells in order to determine their nature. The term **dyskaryosis** refers to the presence of atypical features within cervical epithelial cells, which are predictive of the presence of dysplasia within the ectocervical or endocervical epithelium. Cervical epithelial dysplasia most commonly occurs at the **transformation zone** (the anatomical junction between ectocervical stratified squamous epithelium and endocervical glandular epithelium).

Patients in whom mild dyskaryosis is observed usually undergo repeat cervical smear examination after 6 months, while those with persistent mild dyskaryosis or moderate/severe dyskaryosis undergo detailed examination of the cervix using a colposcope. During this procedure, the cervix is viewed using a magnifying device and biopsies may be taken for histopathological assessment. If an extensive area of cervical dysplasia is identified, the cervical transformation zone may be surgically excised as a cone biopsy, which is a combined diagnostic and potentially curative procedure.

The NHS Breast Screening Programme

Several studies in the 1980s suggested that screening for breast cancer was associated with a significant reduction in mortality from this disease. An NHS-wide screening programme was, therefore,

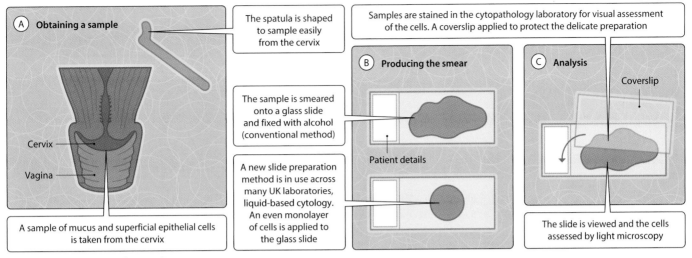

Fig. 3.30.1 The cervical screening programme.

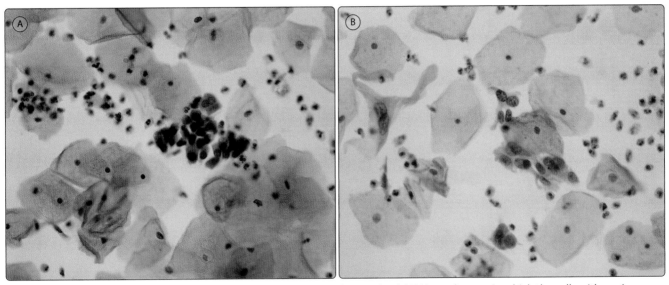

Fig. 3.30.2 Cervical smear preparations stained using the Papanicolou method. (A) Normal smear in which the cells with copious cytoplasm and small regular nuclei are normal ectocervical squamous epithelial cells. The small cluster of cells with less cytoplasm but still with regular nuclei in the centre of the image are normal endocervical columnar cells. (B) Smear showing severe dyskaryosis (predictive of severe dysplasia of the ectocervical squamous epithelium or CIN 3). Normal ectocervical squamous cells are still present but the poorly cohesive collection of dyskaryotic cells close to the centre of the image contain enlarged and irregular nuclei. Scattered individual dyskaryotic cells are also present. Both images also contain neutrophils: small cells with multilobated nuclei. Magnification 400x.

initiated in which women aged 50–64 years (now expanded to 50–70 years) were invited for mammography every 3 years. Individuals in whom an abnormality is detected undergo detailed assessment involving clinical examination, further radiological examination and pathological tests (e.g. fine needle aspiration cytology or needle core biopsy; Ch. 27). The aim is to detect breast cancer at an early stage (i.e. in-situ carcinoma or early small invasive carcinomas) when treatment may be curative.

The aim of detecting breast cancer at an early invasive stage as well as the in-situ stage differs from the Cervical Cancer Screening Programme, which aims to detect cervical cancer primarily at an in-situ (or earlier) stage. However, it is well established that the prognosis of invasive breast cancer is closely linked to tumour size and

that small invasive tumours (especially those <10 mm in size) usually possess a significantly better prognosis than larger tumours.

Screening for non-neoplastic disease

Screening is used for certain inborn errors of metabolism, which, although rare, are potentially catastrophic for affected individuals if not detected early in life. Such diseases include congenital hypothyroidism and phenylketonuria (PKU). Screening involves biochemical examination of blood derived from a pinprick in neonates. Detection during the neonatal period allows successful treatment (e.g. thyroid hormone replacement in hypothyroidism, preventing cretinism, and dietary adjustments in PKU, preventing severe mental retardation).

31. The body at the extremes of age

Questions
- What clinical problems arise in particularly young and particularly old individuals?
- Why is neoplasia generally more common in older people?

Many diseases occur throughout life, but the human body is particularly vulnerable when very young or very old. Many of the conditions affecting individuals at each end of the age spectrum are the same as those occurring throughout life but as well as increased susceptibility to these diseases, these people are at increased risk of developing diseases which are relatively or entirely specific to their age group.

Disease in the very young

Prematurity
Prematurity is associated with particular problems, mainly owing to immaturity of organs and body systems (Fig. 3.31.1). Immaturity leads to increased susceptibility to infection and to less tolerance of changes in local environment as homeostasis is poor.

Congenital malformations
Congenital malformations reflect imperfections in prenatal development and include
- congenital cardiac malformations (Ch. 38)
- cleft lip and/or palate
- spina bifida
- malrotation and/or atresia within the gastrointestinal tract
- club foot (talipes equinovarus).

These may be associated with chromosomal abnormalities. Some congenital malformations are of little or no clinical significance while others (e.g. congenital heart disease, neural tube defects, gastrointestinal tract malformations) may lead to serious consequences including death. Some malformations (e.g. cardiac) may be amenable to treatment while others (e.g. serious neural tube defects) may not be fully or even partially ameliorable even with current therapies. Detailed postmortem examinations may be essential, especially in complex disorders, to enable accurate characterization of the malformation(s) and an assessment of the risk of similar difficulties arising in subsequent pregnancies.

Childhood neoplasia
Children rarely develop tumours characteristically occurring in adults but instead are susceptible to a specific range of neoplasms, many of which are characterized by the presence of 'primitive' or undifferentiated malignant cells (Fig. 3.31.1B). While commonly aggressive when malignant, many of these tumours are nowadays curable with modern therapies.

Other diseases in the young
Small children are at particular risk of infections such as meningitis, pneumonia and septicaemia (i.e. severe infections associated with the presence of bacteria within the blood but without a clinically obvious localized anatomical site for infection) caused by bacteria such as *Neisseria meningitidis* (meningococcus) and *Haemophilus influenzae*. Meningitis remains an unusual but important cause of death into adulthood. Trauma (e.g. road accidents) becomes a dominant cause of morbidity and mortality among adolescents.

Disease in the very old

Degenerative diseases
Elderly individuals commonly develop degenerative diseases simply through 'wear and tear', for example osteoarthritis. Neurodegenerative diseases are a very important cause of morbidity among the elderly since they impair or remove the capability for self-caring and result in the requirement for intermittent or permanent healthcare, with important resource implications for populations with an increasing proportion of elderly members (Fig. 3.31.1C and Ch. 58).

Long-term complications of existing diseases
The elderly are also prone to the complications of disease processes initiating in earlier life such as coronary artery atherosclerosis, leading to ischaemic heart disease and cardiac failure (Ch. 35).

Neoplasia in the elderly
Most neoplasms occurring in adult life show a marked increase in incidence in elderly people, presumably owing to the cumulative effect of environmental exposure to carcinogens and the accumulation of mutations associated with the initiation and progression of neoplasia (Ch. 22). Therapeutic options may be limited in elderly patients developing malignant neoplasms because of the presence of additional disease processes, **comorbidity** (e.g. cardiac or pulmonary disease). This means that a tumour that may be considered technically surgically resectable in a young or middle-aged patient may not be removable in an older patient since the risk of death associated with surgery may be much higher in the latter. Elderly patients may also be more prone to developing adverse effects to other treatments such as radiotherapy and chemotherapy.

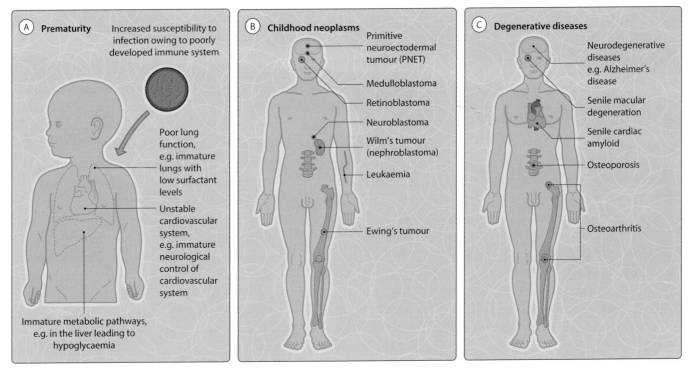

Fig. 3.31.1 Diseases occurring in particular age groups.

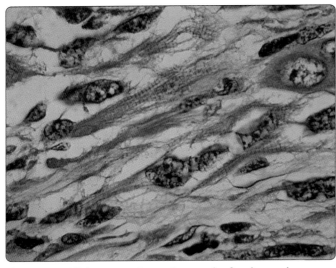

Fig. 3.31.2 High-power photomicrograph of embryonal rhabdomyosarcoma, which is a type of cancer showing striated muscle differentiation (cross-striations). It is usually encountered in children.

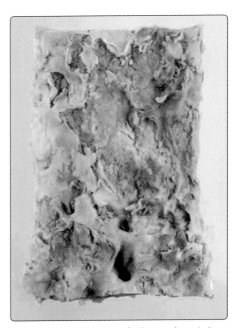

Fig. 3.31.3 A degree of atherosclerosis is present in all elderly individuals in industrialized countries (Ch. 34). This aorta shows confluent ulcerated atherosclerotic plaques.

32. Congenital and inherited diseases

Questions
- What is the difference between congenital and inherited diseases?
- What is the genetic basis underlying disease inheritance?

Congenital diseases are those that are present at birth. Inherited (**familial**) diseases are those passed on from parents via transfer of a genetic defect from parent to offspring. Many inherited diseases are congenital while many congenital diseases are inherited in nature. Congenital malformations are anatomical defects that are present at birth. Many malformations are multifactorial in aetiology, with genetic defects and environmental influences playing variably important roles.

A wide clinical spectrum of congenital and inherited abnormalities exists. The least severe abnormalities may not be clinically apparent or may have relatively inconsequential effects while the most severe forms may be incompatible with life or require early treatment to maximize the chance of survival.

Some inherited syndromes are associated with a specific increased risk of cancer development; these are discussed separately in more detail in Ch. 33.

Table 3.32.1 EXAMPLES OF GENETIC DISEASES

Inheritance pattern and disease	Key clinical features
Autosomal dominant	
Huntington's disease	Progressive neurodegeneration
Neurofibromatosis	Multiple neurofibromas
Familial adenomatous polyposis	Colonic polyps and early colorectal cancer
Polycystic kidney disease	Multiple renal cysts and renal failure
Marfan's syndrome	Tall stature and cardiovascular abnormalities
Familial hypercholesterolaemia	Accelerated atherosclerosis
Autosomal recessive	
Cystic fibrosis	Multisystem including respiratory failure (Ch. 50)
Phenylketonuria	Mental retardation
Glycogen storage diseases	Hypoglycaemia; organ failure
Sickle cell anaemia	Haemolysis and sickle crises
X-linked inheritance pattern	
Duchenne muscular dystrophy	Progressive muscular failure
Haemophilia	Haemorrhage and bruising
Fragile X syndrome[a]	Severe mental retardation

[a]*Approximately 20% of males inheriting the fragile X mutation are phenotypically normal but can act as carriers.*

Diseases with a Mendelian inheritance pattern

Many inherited diseases occur through a mutation within a single gene and with a pattern of inheritance that fits Mendelian genetics. This means that mutations within one or both copies of a gene result in clinical effects with a dominant, codominant or recessive expression pattern (Table 3.32.1 and Fig. 3.32.1). Dominant inheritance means that a mutation within one copy of a gene produces clinical effects when the second gene copy is normal. Recessive inheritance means that mutations are required within both copies of a gene in order that a clinical effect becomes evident. Individuals possessing one recessively inherited mutated gene and one normal gene are termed **carriers**: that is they may pass the mutation to offspring but do not show clinical evidence of the disease. X-linked disorders are those in which a mutation is present within an X-chromosome, usually in a recessive manner; therefore, the effect of the mutation is masked in females whose second gene copy is normal (these individuals are carriers) but is present in males carrying the mutation since there is no second copy of the gene present within the Y-chromosome.

Autosomal dominant diseases

In autosomal dominant diseases, at least one parent will have the disease unless it is occurring as a new mutation. The clinical effect of the genetic mutation may be variable: the degree to which the presence of the mutation produces clinical effect is termed the degree of **penetrance** of the mutation. The clinical effects may be congenital or delayed until later life. For example, Huntington's disease is an incurable progressive neurodegenerative disorder that presents in mid adult life, often after the affected individual has borne offspring.

Autosomal recessive diseases

In autosomal recessive diseases, individuals are only affected if they inherit a mutated gene copy from each parent, who are, therefore, both carriers. According to Mendelian inheritance, there is a 25% chance of offspring inheriting two mutated gene copies if both parents are carriers (Fig. 3.32.1). The majority of recessively inherited diseases affect biochemical pathways and lead to metabolic disturbances. Many present at or soon after birth and require early diagnosis (e.g. glycogen storage diseases, which may lead to neonatal hypoglycaemia) while others require early diagnosis to prevent complications in childhood (e.g. phenylketonuria, which leads to severe mental retardation if untreated) or later life (e.g. familial hypercholesterolaemia, which leads to accelerated atherosclerosis and early-onset ischaemic heart disease if untreated).

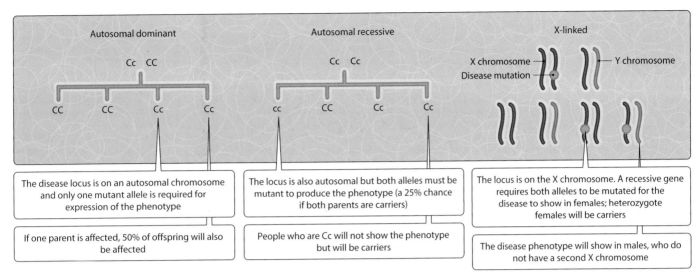

Fig. 3.32.1 Mendelian inheritance of diseases. C, normal gene; c, abnormal gene.

Cystic fibrosis is a good example of a recessively inherited disorder. The disease is caused by a mutation within chromosome 7 (70% of affected individuals possess the ΔF508 mutation), which results in defective chloride ion channels (the cystic fibrosis transmembrane conductance regulator; CFTR) within cell membranes. This results in the production of viscid secretions at several sites within the body and multiple clinical sequelae (Ch. 50). The disease also results in increased sodium chloride concentration within sweat, which forms the basis of a diagnostic test (the sweat test).

X-linked diseases

Individuals with X-linked diseases have mothers who are carriers but who are usually asymptomatic since they possess a second normal gene copy; male and female offspring of maternal carriers have a 50% chance of developing the disease or being mutation carriers, respectively (Fig. 3.32.1).

Diseases with polygenic inheritance

In many diseases, a familial pattern of inheritance is identifiable (i.e. the disease occurs more commonly in relatives of affected individuals that in the general population), indicating a likely genetic component to the aetiology, but the risk of disease development does not follow simple Mendelian inheritance predictions. The contribution of genetic abnormalities to disease development in these cases is probably via the inheritance of mutations within several genes, which individually have low penetrance (i.e. a low likelihood of producing a clinical effect) but which act together to result in a significant genetically determined increase in the risk of disease development. Examples include many congenital malformations (e.g. congenital heart disease occurring outside of the context of a chromosomal disorder), hypertension and schizophrenia.

Chromosomal abnormalities

Congenital abnormalities may result from duplication or loss of all or part of a chromosome and in these circumstances often present as a collection of anomalies that are characteristic of a particular chromosomal abnormality (i.e. a congenital syndrome):

- Down's syndrome: trisomy 21
- Edward's syndrome: trisomy 18
- Patau syndrome: trisomy 13
- Klinefelter syndrome: XXY (most commonly XXY karyotype although Klinefelter syndrome is also manifest in individuals possessing more than two X chromosomes and one or more Y chromosomes)
- Turner's syndrome: XO.

Chromosomal abnormalities are also present in a large number of early spontaneous abortions.

Congenital malformations

Congenital malformations cover a wide spectrum from clinically inconsequential anatomical defects to immediately life-threatening abnormalities. Examples include congenital heart disease (e.g. ventricular septal defect), cleft lip and palate, congenital dislocation of the hip and neural tube defects (e.g. spina bifida).

Causes of congenital malformations

Malformations may occur as a result of a single major 'insult' during embryological development or through a combination of genetic and environmental influences. The latter include diseases present within the mother, infections acquired in utero and the effects of drugs taken by the mother during pregnancy. However, the cause of malformations is unclear in around 50% of cases.

33. Inherited cancer syndromes

Questions
- What forms of cancer result from an inherited predisposition to the disease?
- What are the genetic mechanisms underlying inherited forms of cancer?

Normal human development and the development of disease states are both reliant upon a combination of an individual's genetic composition (nature) and factors within the environment in which the individual exists (nurture). Variations in genetic composition are, therefore, important contributors to disease development.

Genetic mutations and disease development

Neoplastic diseases are characterized by the presence of genetic mutations within the neoplastic tissue (Fig. 3.33.1), which are often multiple in nature and which are associated with loss of the normal mechanisms controlling cellular growth and maturation (Ch. 22). In the majority of cases, cells within the affected individual's non-neoplastic tissue do *not* usually contain demonstrable genetic mutations (i.e. they appear genetically normal).

Inherited predisposition to neoplastic disease

Inherited cancer syndromes are characterized by the presence of a mutation that is inherited from one or both parents and which leads to a significantly increased risk of development of a particular neoplasm or group of neoplasms. This is reflected in an increased incidence of neoplasia within affected families, usually with an identifiable Mendelian pattern of inheritance in a *dominant* fashion (Table 3.33.1). Inherited mutations associated with familial cancer syndromes are usually present within genes important in the regulation of cellular growth and/or maturation and are commonly termed **tumour suppressor genes** (Ch. 22). Neoplasms develop when mutation or loss of the second normal copy of the gene occurs such that the tumour tissue then contains no normal copies of the gene.

Neoplasms occurring within inherited syndromes usually also occur sporadically (i.e. within individuals who have not inherited a genetic mutation) but with different clinicopathological features. For example, neoplasms occurring within an inherited syndrome usually develop at an earlier age and are more commonly multiple. These conditions may be associated with additional non-neoplastic clinical features e.g. familial adenomatous polyposis (Fig. 3.33.2) is associated with abnormal retinal pigmentation termed Roth spots.

Penetrance and familial clustering

Many of the single genetic mutations that are associated with an inherited predisposition to cancer have **high penetrance**. This means that the presence of the genetic mutation usually results in clinically identifiable effects within the affected individual.

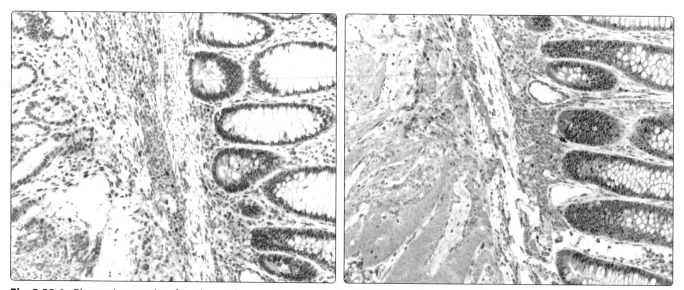

Fig. 3.33.1 Photomicrographs of a colorectal cancer from a patient with the hereditary non-polyposis colorectal cancer (HNPCC) syndrome in which immunohistochemistry shows expression of the DNA mismatch repair enzyme hMLH-1 (brown stain within tumour cell nuclei) but loss of expression of the DNA mismatch repair enzyme hMSH-2 (the negative tumour cell nuclei show only the blue counterstain). In both, the tumour is on the left side and normal large bowel mucosa (serving as an internal positive control for the staining method) is on the right side. This patient has an inherited mutation within the gene encoding hMSH-2.

Table 3.33.1 INHERITED NEOPLASIA SYNDROMES

Syndrome	Gene	Clinical manifestation
Familial adenomatous polyposis	*APC* (adenomatous polyposis coli)	Multiple adenomas in colon and small intestine; colorectal cancer at very young age
Hereditary non-polyposis colorectal cancer	*hMLH-1, hMSH-2, hMSH-6, PMS-1, PMS-2*	Colorectal cancer at young age (especially < 50 years); endometrial carcinoma
Familial breast cancer	*BRCA-1, BRCA-2*	Breast carcinoma at young age (e.g. 20–40 years), may be bilateral; ovarian carcinoma
Multiple endocrine neoplasia (MEN) 1 and 2	*MEN*	Adenomas within endocrine glands; medullary thyroid carcinoma (in MEN 2)
Familial retinoblastoma	*RB1*	Retinoblastoma at young age, often bilateral
Li-Fraumeni syndrome	*p53*	Multiple neoplasms, especially soft tissue sarcomas

However, some genetic mutations do not result in clinical effects as predicted using simple Mendelian inheritance principles alone. In other words, a particular gene may be present but not result in the predicted clinical features; in this situation the gene is termed **low penetrance**.

Familial clustering refers to the observation that some diseases occur at increased frequency within certain families but without a pattern of inheritance that would suggest a single gene is involved. Within neoplasia, colorectal cancer shows familial clustering in 25%. This phenomenon suggests that an inherited (i.e. genetic) predisposition to colorectal cancer exists in these families but that the increased risk is conferred by the inheritance of a collection of several low penetrance genes that collectively act to increase the risk of cancer development.

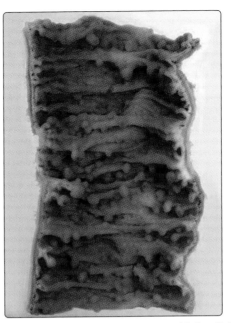

Fig. 3.33.2 Colon from a patient with familial adenomatous polyposis. There are dozens of polyps in this short segment; each polyp is an adenoma.

Pathological characteristics and inherited cancer syndromes

Pathological examination of tumour specimens may reveal characteristics that raise the possibility of an inherited cancer syndrome. For example, colonic adenocarcinoma arising within the hereditary non-polyposis colorectal cancer syndrome more commonly affects the proximal colon and more commonly shows a mucinous growth pattern or poor differentiation on histological examination. Breast cancers occurring in the context of inherited mutations in the *BRCA-1* tend to show features similar to a special subtype of breast cancer termed medullary carcinoma, including increased numbers of mitotic figures. Pathological examination of tissue samples may also provide an indication that an inherited cancer syndrome may be present before cancer develops. For example, examination of colorectal biopsies in familial adenomatous polyposis may reveal the presence of clinically invisible tiny adenomas, termed uni-crypt adenomas.

34. Atherosclerosis

Questions
- What are the key constituents of an atheromatous plaque?
- What are the mechanisms leading to the development of atheroma?
- What are the complications of atherosclerosis?

Atherosclerosis (or atheroma) is an important cause of arterial narrowing. It affects large and medium-sized arteries and is caused by plaques that develop in the intima. In the developed world, atherosclerosis is a common disorder. Its incidence increases with age and it is almost universal in the middle-aged and elderly population.

Morphology

The earliest visible lesion is the fatty streak, a slightly raised yellow spot or band within the intima. These lesions can develop into an atheromatous plaque, which has a soft yellow core covered by a fibrous cap (Fig. 3.34.1). The word atherosclerosis reflects the consistency of the plaques: the soft, lipid-rich core (from the Greek word for porridge, *athere*) and the fibrous sclerotic part. The core consists of necrotic tissue, collections of cholesterol and other lipids, and foam cells containing ingested lipid. Although most of the foam cells are macrophages that derive from blood monocytes, there is evidence that smooth muscle cells can also become phagocytic and transform into foam cells. Around the necrotic core, proliferating smooth muscle cells, macrophages and T-lymphocytes are found. Some lesions also include other inflammatory cells, and chronic inflammation can be important in weakening the plaque or the underlying media. Collagen and other intercellular matrix components are produced by the smooth muscle cells, which act as if they have some characteristics of fibroblasts.

Plaques may undergo a number of changes, in which case they are said to be complicated (Table 3.34.1). Some of these complications have serious sequelae. Stenosis or occlusion of an artery can follow either thrombosis of an ulcerated plaque or haemorrhage into a plaque, with subsequent ischaemia or infarction of the tissue supplied by the artery. Some conditions predispose to the development of critical ischaemia when the normal passage of blood through an artery is prevented:

- reduced oxygen-carrying capacity of the blood, caused either by a low haemoglobin concentration (anaemia) or by irreversible combination of haemoglobin with a substance other than oxygen (e.g. carbon monoxide, which produces carboxyhaemoglobinaemia)
- systemic hypotension, as in shock
- increased oxygen demand by the tissue.

Distal emboli can also cause arterial blockage. There are two types: **thromboemboli** from fragments of thrombus that form on ulcerated plaques, and **cholesterol emboli** composed of necrotic debris from the core of ulcerated plaques.

The inflammatory processes associated with atherosclerosis damage and weaken the wall of the vessel, possibly resulting in aneurysm formation or rupture (Ch. 36 discusses the consequences of atherosclerosis).

Atherosclerosis can affect any artery larger than 2 mm diameter, but in most individuals it tends to affect the aorta, the coronary arteries, the larger arteries of the lower limb, the carotid arteries and the circle of Willis. Aortic atherosclerosis very rarely occludes the lumen of the aorta, but distal emboli and aneurysmal dilatation are common sequelae.

The severity of atheroma in one artery is a poor predictor of its severity elsewhere. Some arteries are rarely affected by atherosclerosis (e.g. the penetrating arteries of the myocardium).

Pathogenesis

The evolving atheromatous plaque is a complex structure in which different components interact with each other. Much of what is known currently can be incorporated into the **response to injury hypothesis**, which proposes that atherosclerosis develops as a chronic inflammatory response to intimal injury. The nature of the initial injury is unclear, but the following factors appear to be involved:

- haemodynamic factors, because atheromatous plaques tend to form where the normal laminar flow of the blood is disturbed (e.g. where arteries branch)
- toxins (e.g. those found in cigarette smoke), which can directly injure the endothelium
- hypertension, which is a known risk factor for atherosclerosis and could act by promoting endothelial cell damage
- hypercholesterolaemia, which can directly impair endothelial cell function.

It has also been suggested that infectious organisms could be a cause of intimal injury; *Chlamydia pneumoniae*, for example, has been isolated from atheromatous plaques.

Once the injury has occurred, monocytes and platelets adhere to the injured endothelium. The monocytes enter the intima where they differentiate into macrophages, and growth factors produced by activated platelets, endothelial cells and macrophages promote proliferation of smooth muscle cells, cause their migration from the media into the intima, and stimulate their production of matrix components such as collagen, elastin and mucopolysaccharides.

The permeability to lipoproteins of the endothelial lining is increased at sites of endothelial damage, and low density lipoproteins (LDL) enter the intima. Some LDL is taken up by macrophages and smooth muscle cells (producing foam cells) while some remains in the extracellular matrix. The lipids are prone to oxidation, and the resulting oxidized LDL is cytotoxic to many different cells, leading to further endothelial cell dysfunction.

Activated macrophages recruit other inflammatory cells and also produce free radicals, which are important in the oxidation of LDL. The lipid-rich core becomes necrotic and attracts more inflammatory cells. Neoangiogenesis occurs with the proliferation of small blood vessels.

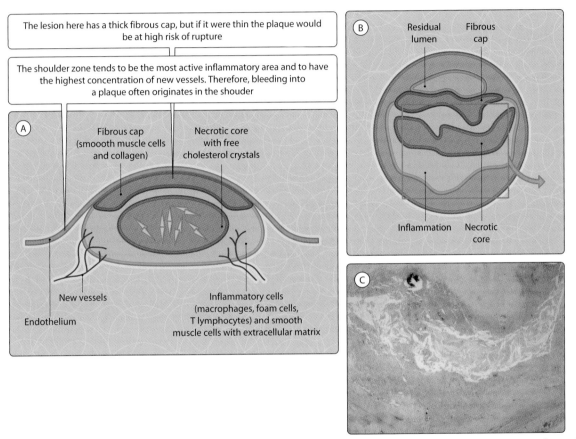

Fig. 3.34.1 An atheromatous plaque. (A) basic structure; (B,C) an atheromatous plaque in a coronary artery shown in a schematic cross-section (B) and as a histological section (C) The rectangle marked in B is the field of view in C.

Table 3.34.1 COMPLICATIONS OF ATHEROSCLEROSIS

Complication	Cause of complication	Possible consequences
Ulceration	Enlarging necrotic core with rupture of fibrous cap	Thrombosis from exposure of thrombogenic material within plaque; cholesterol embolism from release of fragments of necrotic core into the bloodstream
Haemorrhage into plaque	Either rupture of weak blood vessels within the plaque or rupture of the fibrous cap allowing blood to track in from the bloodstream	Narrowing of arterial lumen; weakening of plaque predisposing to (further) rupture
Aneurysmal dilatation	Weakening of the media under the plaque caused by inflammation or ischaemia	Rupture of artery
Calcification	Calcium salt deposition in abnormal tissue of the plaque	No serious clinical sequelae; calcium may render the lesion visible on plain radiographs

35. Ischaemic heart disease

Questions
- What is ischaemic heart disease?
- What are its clinical presentations?
- What are the sequelae and potential complications of myocardial infarction?

Myocardial ischaemia is caused by narrowing of the coronary arteries. The overwhelming cause is atherosclerosis, although there are other, rare, causes (e.g. arteritis, dissecting aneurysm of the aorta, syphilis, or emboli from aortic vegetations). Ischaemic heart disease manifests as angina pectoris, myocardial infarction, sudden death or congestive cardiac failure.

Angina pectoris

Angina pectoris is intermittent chest pain caused by transient, reversible myocardial ischaemia. It is typically experienced as a crushing central chest pain radiating to the left arm or jaw, although the pain can be perceived in many different ways.

In **typical angina**, there is fixed narrowing of the coronary arteries and oxygen supply to the heart is inadequate when the work of the heart increases (e.g. during exercise). Pain occurs on exertion and disappears on resting.

Unstable angina (or crescendo angina) refers to pain occurring with progressively less exertion. The attacks are more severe and last longer. It is thought that it is usually caused by a gradually enlarging thrombus growing on a ruptured plaque. Unstable angina may herald irreversible ischaemic injury (i.e. an infarct).

Prinzmetal angina is caused by a coronary spasm and can occur at rest or during sleep. The aetiology is unclear, but it seems to be linked to atherosclerotic disease, at least in some instances.

Sudden cardiac death

Myocardial hypoxia predisposes to the development of arrhythmias, ventricular fibrillation in particular. The consequence can be sudden collapse and death.

Myocardial infarction

Myocardial infarction is usually caused by complete occlusion of a coronary artery by a thrombus overlying a ruptured plaque. The myocardium exhibits coagulative necrosis, but it takes 8 to 12 hours for this to become visible. In experimental animals, electron microscopy demonstrates ultrastructural changes earlier than this, but these changes are of no use in the practical investigation of a sudden death in clinical circumstances. If death occurs within 8 hours of an infarct, the pathologist will probably find no abnormality of the myocardium at autopsy.

Coronary arteries are end-arteries. The ventricular wall is supplied by perforating branches arising from the epicardial coronary arteries. The subendocardial zone is furthest from the blood supply and it is here that critical ischaemia tends to occur first. As the infarct enlarges, it extends further towards the epicardial surface (Figs 3.35.1 and 3.35.2). The exception is a very narrow band of myocardium immediately adjacent to the endocardium that receives enough oxygen to survive from the blood within the ventricle. The area of infarcted muscle depends on the territory supplied by the obstructed artery. No two hearts are exactly the same, but typical regional infarcts tend to occur in the territories shown in Fig. 3.35.3.

Neutrophils start to infiltrate the necrotic tissue after approximately 12 hours and reach a peak on day 3. Then granulation tissue develops and dominates the picture from approximately week 1 to week 3 as the necrotic muscle is organized. After approximately 3 weeks, increasing fibrosis, progressing from the periphery towards the core of the infarct, represents the conversion of the granulation tissue to a fibrous scar. The scar undergoes remodelling over the ensuing weeks and months as the macrophages disappear and collagen increases (Fig. 3.35.4). The surviving myocardium becomes hypertrophic to compensate, but if muscle loss is extensive the residual myocardium is unable to fully compensate and heart failure results.

Around the edge of the infarct is a zone where the ischaemia is less severe. In this area, the injury is potentially reversible and myocytes may die by apoptosis rather than necrosis (Fig. 3.36.1). The rationale of giving thrombolytic drugs such as streptokinase

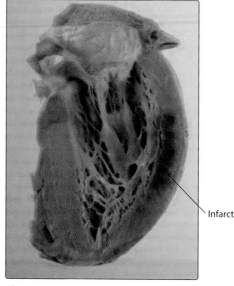

Fig. 3.35.1 Longitudinal section of a heart showing an infarct of the left ventricle.

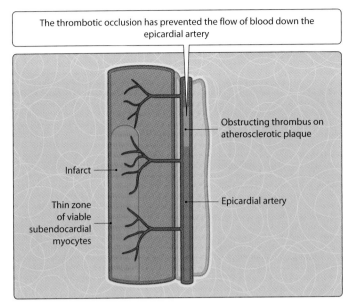

The thrombotic occlusion has prevented the flow of blood down the epicardial artery

Obstructing thrombus on atherosclerotic plaque

Infarct

Epicardial artery

Thin zone of viable subendocardial myocytes

Fig. 3.35.2 Pathogenesis of an infarct (as shown in Fig. 3.35.1).

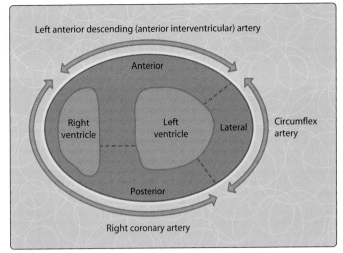

Left anterior descending (anterior interventricular) artery

Anterior

Right ventricle

Left ventricle

Lateral

Circumflex artery

Posterior

Right coronary artery

Fig. 3.35.3 Transverse section through the heart to demonstrate the typical territories of the main coronary arteries.

to patients soon after a myocardial infarct is that some of these injured cells may survive, thus limiting the size of the infarct. However, reperfusion is a two-edged sword because it is associated with the production of highly reactive oxygen species by inflammatory cells, and these free radicals can *cause* death by apoptosis. This is reperfusion injury and it may impede the otherwise beneficial effects of reperfusion in patients with infarcts.

Complications

There are a number of important complications that occur in patients with myocardial infarction.

Arrhythmia. A cause of sudden death.

Rupture of the infarct. Necrotic muscle is weak and can rupture. This is most likely to occur in the first 10 days before fibrosis has become sufficiently established to strengthen the infarct. External rupture through the epicardial surface causes massive haemopericardium and sudden death from tamponade, which is fluid in the pericardium compressing the ventricles and preventing them from filling with blood. Rupture of the interventricular septum causes an acute left-to-right shunt, which may produce congestive cardiac failure.

Papillary muscle dysfunction. Mitral incompetence and acute heart failure can occur when the papillary muscle itself is infarcted or ruptures, or when bulging of the ventricular wall prevents the papillary muscle from holding the mitral valve leaflet in its correct alignment.

Acute pericarditis. Occurs 2–4 days after an infarct and can cause pericardial effusion. A large effusion can cause tamponade.

Mural thrombus. Thrombosis can occur on the endocardial surface overlying an infarct; it is a potential source of systemic thromboembolism.

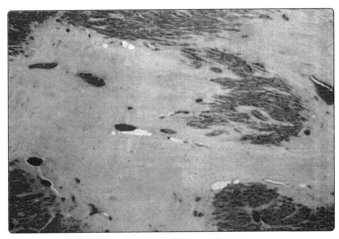

Fig. 3.35.4 Healed myocardial infarct exhibiting mature scar tissue (pale pink) and islands of surviving myocytes (dark pink).

Ventricular aneurysm. This lesion is produced when the weakened left ventricular wall bulges outwards. Ventricular aneurysms are prone to develop mural thrombus.

Pulmonary thromboembolism. The immobility of patients following an acute infarct predisposes to deep venous thrombosis of lower limbs and subsequent pulmonary thromboembolism.

Congestive cardiac failure

In progressive heart failure patchy myocardial fibrosis develops in damaged areas and remaining viable myocardium becomes hypertrophic. Eventually, the left ventricle becomes dilated and the term **ischaemic cardiomyopathy** is sometimes used. There may be a history of anginal chest pain or previous infarction. Death can occur from worsening cardiac failure, arrhythmia or myocardial infarction.

36. Consequences of atherosclerosis and their risk factors

Questions
- What are the clinical sequelae of atherosclerosis apart from ischaemic heart disease?
- What are the risk factors for the development of athero-sclerosis?

The importance of atherosclerosis stems from the serious conditions that can result, principally ischaemic heart disease, cerebral infarction, peripheral vascular disease and aortic aneurysm. Ischaemic heart disease is covered in Ch. 35.

Cerebral infarction

The arteries of the brain are functional end-arteries: that is, the tissue they supply receives blood from that artery alone because the anastomoses between arteries are insufficient to allow for collateral blood supply. As a result, occlusion can cause infarction of the territory supplied by the artery (Fig. 3.36.1). This event can cause a **stroke** (i.e. sudden cerebral dysfunction owing to a vascular event in the brain). Atherosclerosis is the commonest cause of cerebral infarction, either by embolism from a ruptured plaque or by thrombotic occlusion of an atherosclerotic segment (see also Ch. 57).

Aortic aneurysms

An aneurysm is a localized abnormal dilatation of a blood vessel or of the heart. Any condition that weakens the wall of a blood vessel or the heart can produce an aneurysm. Arterial aneurysms are most often caused by atherosclerosis. (Other causes include vasculitis, syphilis, and bacterial infection of the blood vessel wall. The last produces a mycotic aneurysm.)

Atherosclerotic aneurysms occur most frequently in the abdominal aorta, but they can also affect the common iliac arteries and the thoracic aorta. The typical abdominal aortic aneurysm is located between the renal arteries and the aortic bifurcation and is partially filled with thrombus. Complications include obstruction of the ostia of branches of the aorta (e.g. the renal or mesenteric arteries), embolism of thrombotic debris from the aneurysm, and rupture through the weakened wall (Fig. 3.36.2). Rupture is a life-threatening event because of the severe haemorrhage that results; it becomes a significant risk when the aneurysm exceeds 5 cm in diameter and, therefore, surgical repair is likely to be considered in patients who have an aneurysm of this size.

Peripheral vascular disease

The blood supply to the lower limb can be compromised by atherosclerotic narrowing of the arteries. When the collateral circulation becomes inadequate to maintain normal perfusion,

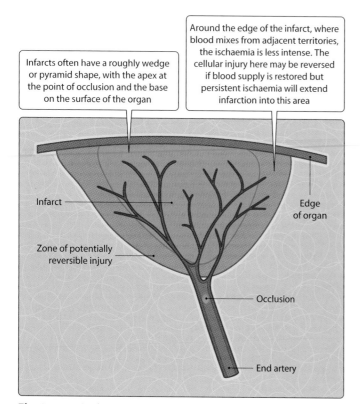

Fig. 3.36.1 Occlusion of an end artery can cause infarction of the territory supplied.

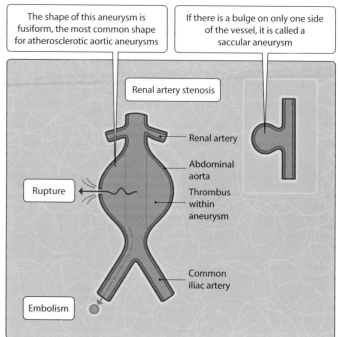

Fig. 3.36.2 A typical aneurysm of the aorta in longitudinal section, showing possible complications.

peripheral vascular disease is the consequence. The ischaemic muscles become painful. In the early stages of the disease, the pain only appears when oxygen demand increases during exercise, and this symptom is called **intermittent claudication**. As the ischaemia worsens, pain is experienced even at rest. Ultimately, the ischaemic tissues become necrotic. Necrosis typically starts at the toes and spreads proximally. **Gangrene** is a common complication; gangrene of the lower extremity is of two types.

Wet gangrene. This is the usual type and is defined as infected necrotic tissue. Morphologically it is characterized by putrefaction: the tissues are discoloured blue or black; there is oedema with blebs of fluid in the skin; and there may be gas production. It normally requires amputation. If untreated by surgery, it is likely to cause death by septicaemia.

Dry gangrene. This is an uncommon event that resembles mummification. The tissues shrink and become waxen in appearance. It occurs in the absence of bacterial infection. However, the risk of putrefaction of the dead tissue by bacteria, with the development of wet gangrene, is a serious risk, so amputation is usually performed.

Epidemiology of atherosclerosis and its risk factors

Atherosclerosis is common in Western countries but less common elsewhere. If individuals from countries with a low incidence migrate to one with a high incidence, their risk of atherosclerosis increases, presumably as a result of adopting a 'Western' lifestyle.

A number of risk factors are known to be important; these can be divided into those that are non-modifiable (e.g. age, sex) and those that are modifiable by lifestyle changes or drug therapy.

Age. The prevalence of atherosclerosis and death rates from the complications of atherosclerosis increase with age.

Male sex. Premenopausal women have a low rate of death from atherosclerosis; the protective factor is thought to be high oestrogen levels. After the menopause, the incidence of complications increases and by old age it equals that of males.

Family history and inherited conditions. A family history of atherosclerotic-related disease confers an increased risk. This familial predisposition is probably polygenic in most cases, but in some patients there is a specific inherited abnormality of lipid metabolism causing hyperlipidaemia. In addition, homocysteinuria, a rare inherited metabolic disorder, carries a markedly increased risk of atherosclerosis.

Hyperlipidaemia. The cholesterol in low density lipoprotein (LDL) is a particularly significant risk factor. The ratio of LDL to high density lipoprotein (HDL) is also important, since a low LDL/HDL ratio appears to have a protective effect. The mechanism is thought to be related to their functions. LDL delivers lipids to tissues, whereas HDL transports it to the liver for metabolism; therefore, HDL could remove lipids from developing plaques. The LDL/HDL ratio is lowered by exercise, consumption of polyunsaturated fatty acids and moderate amounts of alcohol, whereas it is increased by smoking, obesity and a diet rich in saturated fats. Circulating cholesterol can also be reduced by drugs (**statins**).

Hypertension. Raised blood pressure is an important risk factor, and reduction of blood pressure in hypertensive patients reduces their risk of strokes and ischaemic heart disease.

Cigarette smoking. Tobacco can be atherogenic through damage to endothelial cells by circulating toxins, and through the increase in LDL/HDL ratio seen in smokers.

Diabetes mellitus. Diabetic patients are particularly prone to developing atherosclerosis. This important risk factor could act through hypercholesterolaemia or be a direct toxic effect of glucose or its metabolites on endothelial cells.

Obesity. The effects of being overweight are related to the increased incidence of hypertension, diabetes and increased LDL/HDL ratio.

Physical inactivity. Lack of exercise promotes obesity and increases LDL/HDL ratios.

37. Thrombosis and embolism

Questions
- What is the difference between thrombosis and embolism?
- What are the risk factors for thrombosis?
- What may constitute an embolism apart from thrombus?

Insufficiency of blood flow causing tissue ischaemia is one of the most common disease mechanisms encountered in pathology (see Chs 9 and 10). This chapter concentrates on two of the most important causes: thrombosis and embolism.

Thrombosis

A blood clot produced in a blood vessel is called a **thrombus**. It depends on interactions between platelets, the clotting factors of the plasma and the vascular endothelium. Thrombi that form in flowing blood are characterized by the build-up of alternating layers of platelets and fibrin; the result is alternating pale and dark red bands, called lines of Zahn.

There are three main circumstances that predispose to thrombosis. They are known as **Virchow's triad**:
- alterations in the flow of blood
- alterations in the vessel wall
- alterations in the constituents of the blood.

Alterations in the flow of blood include turbulence, which can damage the endothelium, or stagnation, which promotes activation of the clotting cascade. Changes in the vessel wall include anything altering endothelial function (e.g. inflammation) and anatomical abnormalities that could induce turbulent flow. Changes in the constituents of the blood include alterations in viscosity, which tend to promote sludging and stagnation, and abnormalities of the proteins involved in thrombosis and thrombolysis. The last produces a 'hypercoagulable state'; causes include increased oestrogen (pregnancy or contraceptive pill), release of procoagulant factors following surgery or other trauma, the presence of cancer, and inherited conditions such as deficiency in antithrombin III, protein C or protein S.

Thrombi can occur in the chambers of the heart, in arteries or in veins. In the heart, thrombosis can occur on the wall underlying an infarct, in fibrillating atria, within ventricular aneurysms and as a constituent of vegetations. Atherosclerosis is the commonest cause in arteries. In veins, most thrombi probably start in the vicinity of the valves, where turbulent flow occurs. When a vein becomes thrombosed it usually becomes inflamed (**thrombophlebitis**). This should be distinguished from thrombosis in a vein that is already inflamed for some other reason.

Deep venous thrombosis (DVT) is the formation of thrombi in the deep veins of the lower limb and pelvis. It is a common clinical problem, and its importance lies in the complication of pulmonary embolism (see below) that can follow. This is a feared complication of major surgery, since postoperative patients are at increased risk of DVT. Therefore, postoperative patients receive prophylaxis to reduce the risk of thrombosis. The factors that contribute to DVT in the postoperative patient can be understood by applying the principles of Virchow's triad:
- alteration in blood flow through the veins: poor flow is seen in immobile or bedridden patients
- changes in the wall of the vein: irritation or trauma of the veins may occur, especially during pelvic or lower limb surgery
- hypercoagulability of the blood: an increased tendency to thrombus formation (e.g. from trauma of surgery).

There are several possible sequelae of thrombosis (Fig. 3.37.1):
- complete resolution with disappearance of the thrombus through the thrombolytic mechanisms and restoration of normal anatomy
- organization of the thrombus by granulation tissue, producing a fibrous scar that causes stenosis or occlusion
- embolism by fragments of thrombus breaking off into the circulation.

Embolism

An embolus is an object that is carried through the circulation to a site distant from its point of origin. Essentially, the object reaches an area where it is too big to get any further and becomes stuck. The clinical significance stems mainly from the obstruction to blood flow. Many materials can embolize.

Thromboembolism. Thrombus is by far the commonest source of embolism.

Cholesterol embolism. Ulcerated atheromatous plaques can liberate fragments of their necrotic cholesterol-rich cores into the circulation. These are cholesterol (or atheromatous) emboli (Fig. 3.37.2).

Fat embolism. This event is seen after trauma, especially bone fractures and burns. Sometimes, fragments of fatty marrow may embolize. A more common source of fat embolism is coalescence of serum lipid into globules that block the circulation. Symptoms start 1–3 days after injury and typically include breathlessness, neurological symptoms, petechial rash and thrombocytopenia, which result from involvement of the lungs, brain, skin and platelets, respectively.

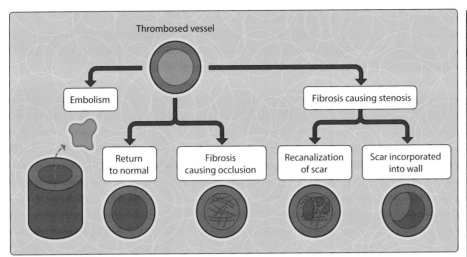

Fig. 3.37.1 Sequelae of intravascular thrombosis.

Thrombosed vessel

Embolism

Fibrosis causing stenosis

Return to normal

Fibrosis causing occlusion

Recanalization of scar

Scar incorporated into wall

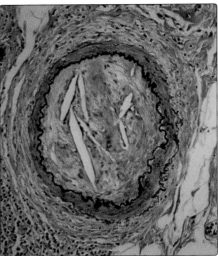

Fig. 3.37.2 Healing cholesterol embolus in a branch of the superior mesenteric artery. The embolism originated from an ulcerated atheromatous plaque in the aorta. This patient had small bowel ischaemia as a result of multiple cholesterol emboli. The cleft-like spaces represent the site of cholesterol crystals. Elastic van Gieson stain.

Gas embolism. There are two main circumstances in which gas bubbles obstruct the circulation and cause ischaemia:

- nitrogen bubbles: if a diver who has been breathing air under pressure at depth ascends too quickly, nitrogen can come out of solution producing bubbles in the blood; the symptoms were common before the use of decompression schedules became routine, and include the bends (painful joints), the chokes (respiratory distress), the staggers (central nervous symptoms) and the itch (a rash).
- air: quantities of air sufficient to cause symptoms can occasionally enter via the veins of the neck and thorax during trauma, or the uterine veins during traumatic birth.

Amniotic fluid embolism. This rare but serious complication of labour follows fluid entry via ruptured uterine veins.

Tumour embolism. Fragments of tumour within vessels can become detached and embolize.

Foreign bodies. On rare occasions, foreign bodies such as catheter tips and bullets can embolize. In drug addicts, talc injected into the veins along with the active drug can be found in small vessels (Fig. 3.37.3).

The clinical effects of emboli depend on whether the systemic or pulmonary circulation is involved.

Pulmonary embolus. With rare exceptions, clinically significant pulmonary emboli are thromboemboli from DVT. The thromboembolus passes into the right side of the heart and enters the pulmonary arteries. Large thromboemboli occlude

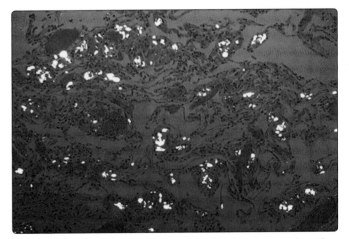

Fig. 3.37.3 Talc in small pulmonary vessels. Arterioles and capillaries contain crystals that display birefringence under polarized light. This material was injected into a vein by a drug abuser.

the pulmonary trunk and cause sudden death through acute circulatory failure. Small pulmonary thromboemboli are usually asymptomatic, but they can cause infarction of lung tissue and, if numerous, can cause pulmonary hypertension.

Systemic embolus. The commonest source of a systemic embolus is a thrombus within the heart or great vessels. The most important sites for embolization are the lower limbs and the brain. On very rare occasions, a venous thromboembolus passes into the systemic circulation through a patent foramen ovale; this occurrence is called paradoxical embolism.

38. Valvular and congenital heart disease

Questions
- What are the main clinical effects of cardiac valvular disease?
- What is rheumatic fever?
- What are the most common forms of congenital heart disease?

This chapter considers some diseases associated with abnormal patterns of flow through the heart.

Valvular heart disease

The significance of valvular heart disease is twofold: impairing normal function and increasing the risk of valve infection.

If **normal valve function** is impaired, there can be narrowing (stenosis), regurgitation (incompetence) or both, depending on the morphological abnormality. Disease of the heart may follow. For example, a stenotic aortic valve requires extra effort on the part of the left ventricle to expel blood (i.e. there is pressure overload). If the aortic valve is incompetent, part of the ejection fraction regurgitates back into the left ventricle, so the ventricle must work harder to maintain cardiac output (i.e. there is volume overload). Pressure or volume overload will lead to left ventricular hypertrophy and ultimately to heart failure. If both are present, the risk of heart failure is compounded. Cardiac valve abnormalities are also associated with sudden unexpected death.

There is also an increased risk of **infective endocarditis** as any anatomical abnormality makes the valve susceptible to infection by bacteria or other organisms circulating in the blood; infection rarely develops on normal valves. Injury to a mucosal surface can cause bacteria to enter the bloodstream (bacteraemia); for example, mouth commensal bacteria can enter the bloodstream following dental treatment or even brushing the teeth; *Streptococcus viridans* is the organism most often responsible in these circumstances. On other occasions, the source is intravenous drug abuse with injection of contaminated material. A characteristic feature of infective endocarditis is the formation of **vegetations** on the valves: irregular deposits of fibrin, platelets and bacteria.

Causes of valvular heart disease

A wide variety of diseases affect the heart valves. Some occur as congenital malformations (see below) while others are acquired.

Rheumatic fever can lead to valvular heart disease (**chronic rheumatic heart disease**). Rheumatic fever is an autoimmune condition in which inflammation of many organs follows an episode of pharyngitis caused by group A streptococci. It appears that antibodies directed against the streptococci cross-react with normal proteins present in the heart, joints and other tissues. Inflammation of the heart in rheumatic fever is called **acute rheumatic carditis**. When the valves are involved, vegetations form on them; these are smaller than the vegetations typical of infective endocarditis and do not contain bacteria. Healing occurs with scar formation; the fibrosis can cause stenosis by reducing the valve diameter and/or regurgitation by preventing proper closure of the valve leaflets.

Calcification of the aortic valve often occurs with ageing. Sometimes, the calcified leaflets become so rigid that clinically apparent stenosis occurs (**calcific aortic stenosis**). Although calcification is often seen in normal valves, it is more common in **congenitally bicuspid aortic valves**, a common lesion in which the aortic valve is composed of two leaflets instead of three.

The mitral valve can also be affected, leading to **mitral regurgitation**. Mitral regurgitation can occur in many different circumstances, including dilated valve rings in cardiac failure, papillary muscle dysfunction or rupture following myocardial infarction, and chronic rheumatic heart disease. However, the most common cause of isolated mitral regurgitation is **mitral valve prolapse**, sometimes called floppy mitral valve, caused by myxoid degeneration of the valve leaflets.

Congenital heart disease

Anomalous embryological development of the heart is the commonest cause of childhood heart disease in industrialized countries. In some of those affected, environmental factors such as congenital rubella infection are responsible. In others, a genetic factor can be identified. However, in most the cause is unknown.

There are many different types of congenital heart disease and they often occur in combination. They can be classified functionally as left-to-right shunts, right-to-left shunts, and obstructions. All congenital anomalies increase the risk of infective endocarditis. Most of them also predispose to arrhythmias and carry a risk of sudden cardiac death.

Left-to-right shunts

Left-to-right shunts are the commonest type. They are defects that allow blood to flow from the high-pressure left circulation to the low-pressure right circulation, and include atrial septal defect (ASD), ventricular septal defect (VSD) and patent ductus arteriosus. ASD and VSD are holes that allow blood to pass through the interatrial and interventricular septa, respectively; they are the commonest congenital heart anomalies. The ductus arteriosus connects the pulmonary artery to the aorta. It normally constricts in the first day of life and becomes completely occluded in the first few months, but if this process fails, a persistent connection remains between the right and left arterial trees.

Left-to-right shunts are usually asymptomatic or associated with only mild symptoms during childhood (although large defects can cause early cardiac failure owing to volume overload). However, pulmonary hypertension results from the increased volume of blood flowing through the lungs and by late childhood or early adulthood the pressure in the pulmonary circulation approaches systemic levels. At this point, the direction of the shunt is reversed and flow becomes bidirectional or right to left. As a result, unoxygenated blood from the right circulation mixes with oxygenated blood and the patient becomes cyanotic, with worsening symptoms of breathlessness and fatigue. Eventually, heart failure occurs. This combination of pulmonary hypertension and heart failure as a consequence of shunt reversal is called **Eisenmenger syndrome** (Fig. 3.38.1).

Right-to-left shunts

The cardinal feature of right-to-left shunts is cyanosis at or soon after birth. Indeed, the term cyanotic congenital heart disease is often applied to them. The commonest is **tetralogy of Fallot**, which comprises:

- a VSD
- an aortic root that overrides the VSD
- right ventricular outflow obstruction caused by a narrow pulmonary artery and/or valve
- right ventricular hypertrophy.

The right ventricular outflow obstruction causes high pressure in the right ventricle, which becomes hypertrophic. The high right ventricular pressure pushes blood through the VSD, so unoxygenated blood joins blood in the systemic circulation, causing cyanosis (Fig. 3.38.2).

Congenital obstructive lesions

Many different stenotic lesions of the valves or great vessels have been described. The most common are **congenital aortic valve stenosis** and **coarctation of the aorta**. Both can produce heart failure through pressure overload and other complications. Coarctation of the aorta can be pre- or postductal.

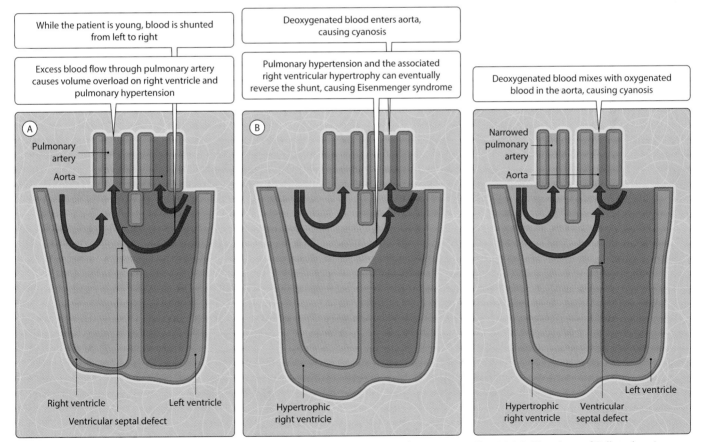

Fig. 3.38.1 Flow through the ventricles in the heart of a patient with a ventricular septal defect. (A) While the patient is young; (B) shunt reversal occurring over time (Eisenmenger syndrome). Oxygenated blood, red; deoxygenated blood, blue; direction of flow, arrows.

Fig. 3.38.2 Tetralogy of Fallot, showing ventricular septal defect, right ventricular hypertrophy, over-riding aorta and narrowing of pulmonary outflow.

39. Cardiomyopathies and dissecting haematoma of the aorta

Questions
- What is a cardiomyopathy and what are the most common causes?
- How may cardiomyopathies present clinically?
- What is a dissecting haematoma of the aorta and what are its complications?

Cardiomyopathies

The term cardiomyopathy does not have a precise definition, but it is generally used to describe three conditions: hypertrophic, dilated and restrictive cardiomyopathy. Dilated cardiomyopathy is the commonest.

Dilated cardiomyopathy

The definition of dilated cardiomyopathy (also known as congestive cardiomyopathy) is progressive cardiac hypertrophy with dilatation affecting all chambers and associated with progressive systolic dysfunction. It is caused by diffuse damage to the myocardium and can have a number of aetiologies, including:

- viral infections, e.g. coxsackievirus B
- drugs and toxins, e.g. alcohol abuse
- hereditary abnormalities of cytoskeletal proteins.

The systolic dysfunction produces heart failure, which is often fatal. In some cases, mural thrombi form in the flabby cardiac chambers. If they break off, they give rise to embolic complications.

Hypertrophic cardiomyopathy

This condition is characterized by a hypertrophic left ventricle that can contract strongly, but it is stiff and diastolic filling is impaired. This stiffness is more precisely described as reduced ventricular compliance. A number of different genetic defects can produce this condition; the genes involved code for a variety of sarcomeric proteins. Although some cases arise sporadically, approximately half of patients inherit the condition as an autosomal dominant trait with variable penetrance and expression. There are a number of clinical features (Fig. 3.39.1):

- **heart failure**, which can result from the diastolic dysfunction of the thick, rigid ventricle, or from ventricular outflow obstruction during systole; the latter results from the narrow gap between the anterior mitral valve leaflet and the hypertrophic interventricular septum
- **ischaemic heart disease**, which occurs because the hypertrophic mass of muscle requires a large blood supply; angina can occur even in the absence of coronary artery stenosis
- **arrhythmia and sudden death**.

Note that hypertrophic cardiomyopathy is a specific disease caused by genetic defects in sarcomeric proteins. It is not to be confused with the concept of left ventricular hypertrophy in general.

Restrictive cardiomyopathy

Several pathological processes can produce restrictive cardiomyopathy, which is characterized by a stiff ventricle (diminished ventricular compliance) and impaired ventricular filling during diastole. Like hypertrophic cardiomyopathy, symptoms result from diastolic failure. Unlike that condition, however, systole is not hyperdynamic. Indeed, there may also be systolic dysfunction in restrictive cardiomyopathy if contractility is affected. Causes include:

- endomyocardial fibrosis, a disease of unknown cause in which the endocardium exhibits fibrous thickening
- amyloidosis
- haemochromatosis.

Although restrictive cardiomyopathy is rare in developed countries, restrictive cardiomyopathy caused by endomyocardial fibrosis accounts for approximately 10% of childhood heart disease in the tropics.

Dissecting haematoma of the aorta

If blood enters the wall of the aorta through a tear, it tends to track longitudinally along the bundles of collagen and elastin in the tunica media. The common name for this condition used to be a dissecting aneurysm, but the lesion is not aneurysmal in the true sense because the aorta is not dilated, and so the preferred name is now dissecting haematoma.

The initiating event is a tear in the aortic intima that allows blood to enter the media. In most cases, this tear is within 10 cm of the aortic valve (Fig. 3.39.2). Next, blood is forced along the media by the blood pressure, usually along the junction between the middle two-thirds and outer one-third of the media. There are a number of serious consequences of aortic dissection, as illustrated in Fig. 3.39.3. If untreated, survival is likely only if the blood reenters the aorta through a second intimal tear, producing a double-barrelled aorta. This event allows blood to rejoin the aortic lumen after flowing through the dissection, but it is a rare occurrence. The causes of aortic dissection are:

- hypertension
- weakness of the tunica media
- iatrogenic.

Hypertension is probably the most common cause. The risk of aortic dissection increases as the blood pressure rises.

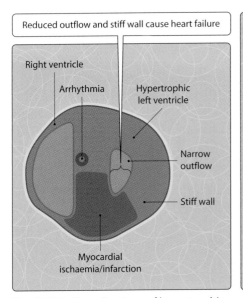

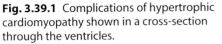

Reduced outflow and stiff wall cause heart failure

Right ventricle

Arrhythmia

Hypertrophic left ventricle

Narrow outflow

Stiff wall

Myocardial ischaemia/infarction

Fig. 3.39.1 Complications of hypertrophic cardiomyopathy shown in a cross-section through the ventricles.

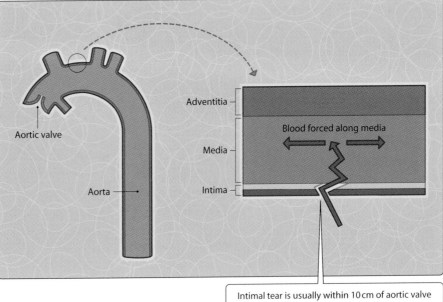

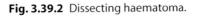

Aortic valve

Aorta

Adventitia

Blood forced along media

Media

Intima

Intimal tear is usually within 10 cm of aortic valve

Fig. 3.39.2 Dissecting haematoma.

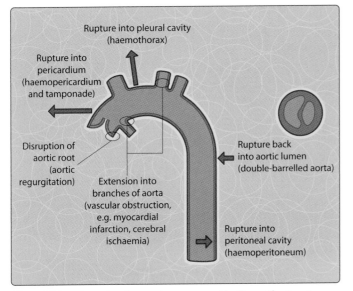

Rupture into pleural cavity (haemothorax)

Rupture into pericardium (haemopericardium and tamponade)

Disruption of aortic root (aortic regurgitation)

Extension into branches of aorta (vascular obstruction, e.g. myocardial infarction, cerebral ischaemia)

Rupture back into aortic lumen (double-barrelled aorta)

Rupture into peritoneal cavity (haemoperitoneum)

Fig. 3.39.3 Dissecting haematoma: complications. The inset shows a cross-section through a double-barrelled aorta.

Weakness of the tunica media is an important factor in certain congenital abnormalities of the connective tissues. For example, **Marfan syndrome** is an inherited abnormality of fibrillin 1, and a consequence of this condition is weakness of the aortic wall predisposing to dissecting haematoma. However, medial weakness in the general population is more controversial: histological changes known as **cystic medial degeneration** have been described in the aortas of patients with aortic dissection whether they have Marfan syndrome or not, and it has been thought that this finding represents an underlying weakness of the aortic wall. However, cystic medial degeneration can also be observed in aortas from otherwise normal individuals and the significance of these appearances is unclear.

Cannulation of the aorta with a catheter can damage the intima, causing an iatrogenic, dissecting haematoma.

Presentation and treatment

Dissecting haematoma can present in several ways:

- sudden, severe pain in chest and back, which may move downwards as dissection propagates
- if branches of the aorta are stenosed, there will be ischaemia of the organs supplied
- sudden collapse if external rupture occurs into the pericardium, pleural space or peritoneum
- acute insufficiency of the aortic valve if the aortic root is disrupted.

The treatment is first to reduce the blood pressure, which typically rises even higher than usual in these patients as a result of pain and stress, and second to operate, if possible, to repair the defect.

40. Heart failure

Questions
- What are the most common causes of heart failure?
- What are the clinical sequelae of heart failure?

Heart failure is the clinical syndrome that results when the heart is unable to pump enough blood to supply the metabolic needs of the body. Cardiogenic shock (Ch. 13) is a type of heart failure. However, in clinical practice, the term heart failure tends to be used for chronic conditions, while cardiogenic shock implies acute pump failure. Heart failure can be thought of conceptually in a number of different ways that help to explain the mechanism of failure.

Backward failure and forward failure

Heart failure can be considered as either backward or forward in type. Backward heart failure describes the condition in which the ventricle is unable to discharge its contents properly during systole, resulting in an increase in end-diastolic volume. The volume and pressure in the atrium behind the failing ventricle rise, and the pressure in the venous and capillary beds behind the ventricle increases. In a sense, the blood 'dams up' behind the failing ventricle. The congestive features of heart failure (see below) can be explained by this hypothesis.

The concept of forward heart failure describes inadequate delivery of blood to the arterial system because of reduced cardiac output, so organs are inadequately perfused: reduced perfusion of skeletal muscles causes fatigue; reduced perfusion of the extremities causes them to be cold and pale; and underperfusion of the kidneys causes fluid retention in part by a reduction in glomerular filtration rate and in part by activation of the renin–angiotensin–aldosterone system. The fluid retention contributes to the heart failure by increasing the plasma volume, thus increasing the metabolic demands on the myocardium.

Diastolic and systolic failure

Concepts of diastolic and systolic failure are useful in thinking about what is happening in the heart itself. In diastolic failure, the ability of the heart to accept blood is impaired because of failure of normal ventricular relaxation (e.g. in hypertrophic cardiomyopathy, amyloidosis and restrictive cardiomyopathy). Insufficient blood enters the ventricle during diastole so end-diastolic volume is low. Even if most of this blood is expelled by a strongly contracting myocardium, the cardiac output will be low. In systolic failure, blood enters the ventricle normally but the ejection fraction is low because the muscle does not contract forcefully. Again, the result is a low cardiac output.

Although *pure* examples of systolic and diastolic dysfunction occur, in most patients both types coexist. For example, consider the pathophysiology in a patient with a previous large myocardial infarction that has been replaced by a scar. Diastolic dysfunction may occur because the scarred myocardium is not distensible and so the capacity of the myocardium to accept blood is reduced. However, there may also be systolic failure caused by loss of contractile myocardium in the scarred area.

Left-sided and right-sided failure

Cardiac failure may affect the left, the right or both ventricles. Congestive symptoms initially localize behind the affected ventricle, consistent with the backward failure hypothesis. Thus, in left-sided failure, pulmonary congestion and oedema predominate. The chronic pulmonary congestion causes raised pulmonary arterial pressure, and eventually the right ventricle also fails. Indeed, the commonest cause of right ventricular failure is left ventricular failure.

In right-sided heart failure, congestion of the systemic veins causes congestion and enlargement of the spleen and liver (in the latter, chronic passive venous congestion produces the classic pathological appearance on the cut surfaces of 'nutmeg liver'). Right ventricular failure also causes oedema of the soft tissues, and effusions in the pleural, pericardial and abdominal cavities.

Compensated and decompensated failure

As the heart begins to fail, compensatory mechanisms initially maintain cardiac output. This is the phase of compensated heart failure. The mechanisms involved include:

- increased sympathetic drive, causing more forceful contraction (inotropic effect) and increased heart rate
- remodelling of the heart, with dilatation (which increases myocyte length, increasing the force of contraction according to Starling's law of the heart) and hypertrophy (which increases the mass of heart muscle)
- fluid retention in the kidneys, causing increased plasma volume.

However, the inotropism, tachycardia, hypertrophy and increased plasma volume all increase the oxygen requirements of the already compromised myocardium. Moreover, hypertrophic myocardium is more prone to ischaemia than normal myocardium, because when ventricular myocardium becomes hypertrophic the density of capillaries decreases and the ratio of capillaries to myocytes is reduced. Furthermore, the hypertrophic muscle is stiffer than normal and the hypertrophic ventricles do not fill normally, causing diastolic dysfunction. With time, the function of the myocardium gradually diminishes until the heart cannot provide a cardiac output sufficient for the needs of the body. When this point is reached, the heart failure is decompensated. Initially, the decompensation is only evident during exercise, when the systemic blood flow is increased, but eventually the features become apparent even at rest. There is also an increased risk of ventricular arrhythmias, which are an important cause of sudden death in these patients.

Causes of heart failure

Causes of heart failure can be divided into three main groups.

Ventricular overload. The ventricle is required to meet an increased mechanical load, either because it has to cope with an excessive volume of blood or with an increased resistance in the arterial tree. The former produces volume overload or increased preload, and the latter produces pressure overload or increased afterload. Causes are hypertension, causing left ventricular failure through increased afterload; and valvular heart disease, regurgitant valves increasing preload, stenotic valves increasing afterload.

Cardiac muscle function. The cardiac muscle function is impaired, as in ischaemic heart disease, myocarditis and dilated cardiomyopathy.

Heart filling. The filling of the heart is restricted, for example in mitral or tricuspid stenosis, cardiac tamponade, constrictive pericarditis, hypertrophic cardiomyopathy, restrictive cardiomyopathy, and cardiac amyloid.

In industrialized countries, ischaemic heart disease and systemic hypertension are the commonest causes of heart failure. Valvular heart disease is another common cause. Occasionally, an unusually high cardiac output can precipitate heart failure. Such high-output states include thyrotoxicosis, anaemia, arteriovenous fistula and Paget disease of the bone.

The morphological changes in the heart are related to the mechanisms of the heart failure. Examples are shown in Fig. 3.40.1.

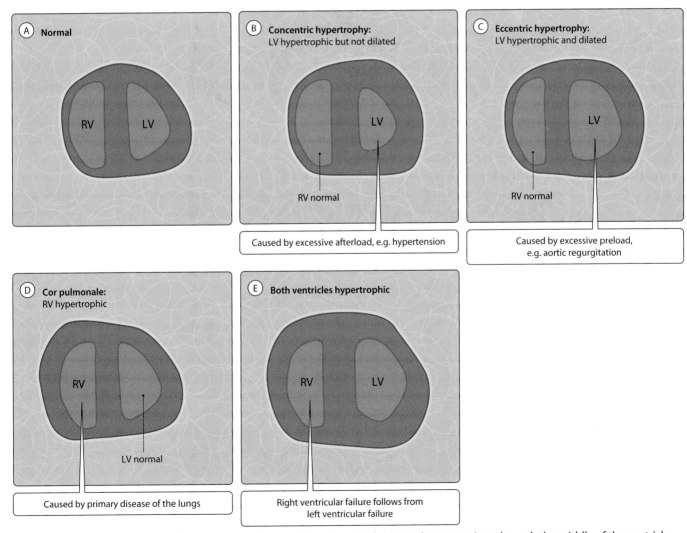

Fig. 3.40.1 Common patterns of hypertrophy in the ventricles shown in horizontal cross-sections through the middle of the ventricles. LV, left ventricle; RV, right ventricle.

41. Hypertension and hypertensive heart disease

Questions
- What are the main risk factors for hypertension?
- What changes are seen in the heart and blood vessels in hypertension?
- What are the pathological mechanisms involved in the development of hypertension?

Pathological increases in blood pressure can affect the systemic or pulmonary circulation and may be seen in the arteries or veins. Hypertension of the systemic arteries is covered here. It is a common health problem and is a risk factor for diseases that include atheroma, heart failure, aortic dissection and renal failure. Studies have shown that the risk of these complications increases as the blood pressure rises, and that antihypertensive treatment reduces the morbidity and mortality.

The **definition of high blood pressure** is arbitrary in that blood pressure exhibits a Gaussian distribution so there is no clear boundary between hypertension and normal blood pressure. In general, hypertension is commonly defined as a systolic blood pressure of 140 mmHg or greater or a diastolic blood pressure of 90 mmHg or greater.

If untreated, hypertension can progress to **malignant hypertension**, which is defined as markedly elevated blood pressure (diastolic pressure usually >120 mmHg). It is associated with rapid progression of target organ disease (e.g. renal failure and retinal damage).

Vascular changes in hypertension

The principal effect of hypertension in **large** and **medium-sized arteries** is to accelerate the development of atheroma. By comparison, **arterioles** exhibit two different kinds of morphological change in hypertension.

Hyaline arteriolosclerosis. This is an ageing-related change common in elderly individuals. However, it appears earlier in patients with either hypertension or diabetes. It is characterized by hyaline thickening of the walls of arterioles, with some luminal narrowing. It is believed to be caused by leakage of plasma proteins into the wall and increased production of extracellular matrix by smooth muscle cells in response to raised blood pressure.

Hyperplastic arteriolosclerosis. This condition is seen in more severe hypertension, including malignant hypertension. It is characterized by proliferation of smooth muscle cells and basement membrane material, causing concentric laminations. The result is progressive, severe narrowing of the lumen.

Regulation of normal blood pressure

Blood pressure is a function of cardiac output and peripheral resistance. Cardiac output is affected by the intravascular volume, while the peripheral resistance is controlled principally by arteriolar tone (Fig. 3.41.1).

The kidney has a central role in blood pressure regulation through the renin–angiotensin–aldosterone system and the glomerular filtration rate, which is why so many renal diseases are associated with hypertension. The juxtaglomerular apparatus of the kidney responds to reduced blood pressure by secreting renin, which converts angiotensinogen into angiotensin I, which is converted by angiotensin-converting enzyme (ACE) into angiotensin II. Angiotensin II acts to increase blood pressure in two ways: by increasing peripheral resistance and by stimulating production of aldosterone, which increases intravascular volume by increasing renal absorption of salt and water. In addition, any reduction in glomerular filtration rate reduces sodium excretion and tends to increase blood pressure.

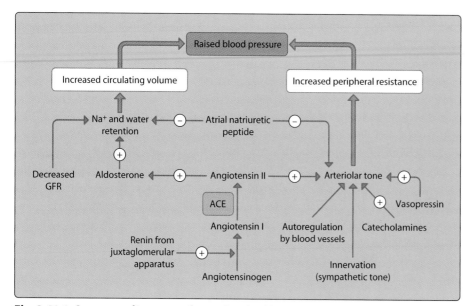

Fig. 3.41.1 Summary of important factors involved in maintaining blood pressure. ACE, angiotensin-converting enzyme; GFR, glomerular filtration rate.

Another factor affecting blood pressure is atrial natriuretic peptide, which is secreted by the cardiac atria in response to volume expansion. It reduces blood pressure by decreasing renal absorption of salt and water and causing vasodilation.

Pathogenesis of hypertension

Between 5 and 10% of patients have an identifiable cause of their hypertension and are said to have secondary hypertension. The other 90–95% of patients have no specific cause and are said to have essential hypertension.

Essential hypertension

The current concept of essential hypertension is that it represents a collection of inherited genetic conditions modified by environmental factors. The inherited contribution appears to be polygenic and leads to clustering in families. Environmental factors shown to be associated with high blood include high sodium intake, reduced calcium and potassium intake, obesity, smoking, stress, high ethanol intake and lack of physical exercise.

One model of essential hypertension proposes that the initiating event is increased circulating volume, resulting in raised cardiac output. Patients with essential hypertension appear to have lower rates of sodium excretion, in keeping with this hypothesis. An alternative idea is that the initiating event is chronic vasoconstriction of arterioles, leading to permanent structural changes in their walls, thus increasing peripheral resistance.

Secondary hypertension

The mechanisms producing secondary hypertension can be understood by the effects of the aetiological factors on the homeostatic processes that control blood pressure.

Renal artery stenosis. Reduced blood flow to the kidney decreases glomerular filtration and stimulates renin release. In older patients, the stenosis is usually caused by atheroma of the ostium of the renal artery where it arises from the aorta. In younger patients, fibromuscular anomalies causing narrowing of the renal artery are most frequent. Vasculitis is another cause.

Diseases of the renal parenchyma. For example, glomerulonephritis, polycystic disease and diabetic nephropathy can all be associated with abnormalities in renal control of blood pressure and are common causes of hypertension.

Endocrine dysfunction. Some hormones have effects on peripheral resistance and/or renal function. For example, tumours that secrete catecholamines (phaeochromocytomas) or mineralocorticoids (adrenocortical adenomas) produce hypertension. Excess glucocorticoids, as seen in steroid therapy or Cushing's syndrome, also cause blood pressure to rise.

Sleep apnoea. This is a fairly common cause of hypertension. The typical patient is obese and prone to stop breathing for periods of up to a minute or more while asleep. The pathogenesis of hypertension is not clear but could be related to the increased sympathetic activity, and hence increased cardiac output and peripheral vascular resistance, associated with chronic hypoxia.

Effects of hypertension on the heart

The definition of **hypertensive heart disease** is left ventricular hypertrophy in a hypertensive individual, provided other causes of left ventricular hypertrophy have been excluded. The hypertrophy is a response to the increased functional demand on the heart muscle as it pumps against an increased pressure load. The principal complications are ischaemic heart disease and heart failure (Fig. 3.41.2). Several mechanisms combine to produce ischaemic heart disease in these patients:

- the hypertrophic myocardium has increased oxygen requirements
- in pathological hypertrophy, the capillaries do not multiply at a rate sufficient to maintain the normal density of capillaries in the myocardium, so the blood supply to the enlarged myocardium is insufficient for normal perfusion
- the hypertension predisposes to atheromatous disease of the coronary arteries.

Left ventricular failure can arise from reduced compliance of the myocardium, which occurs as result of increased stiffness of the thickened muscle. The consequence is diastolic dysfunction, with failure of normal filling during diastole. In addition, ischaemia can contribute to heart failure.

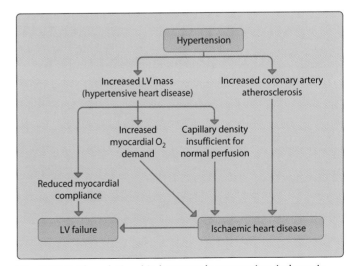

Fig. 3.41.2 The relationship between hypertension, ischaemic heart disease and left ventricular failure. LV, left ventricle.

42. Pneumonia

Questions
- What is pneumonia?
- What are the clinical and pathological features of pneumonia?

The term pneumonia is most commonly used to indicate the presence of a lung infection. However, pneumonia can also sometimes be used to refer to other forms of inflammatory lung disease that interfere with lung function but are not necessarily associated with the presence of an infective organism within the lung. Pneumonia is classically associated with bacterial infection, which most commonly takes the form of acute inflammation involving the alveolar spaces. However, some forms of pneumonia predominantly involve the alveolar walls (**interstitial pneumonia**). Inflammation may spread to involve the pleura (**pleurisy**) or pericardium (**pericarditis**) and bacteria may enter the bloodstream (**septicaemia**) and travel to other organs (e.g. resulting in a cerebral abscess).

Infections within the lung

Lung tissue is exposed to many pathogens within inhaled air and may become infected with a wide range of microorganisms (Table 3.42.1). Bacteria are the organisms most commonly associated with the development of pneumonia, with certain types particularly characteristic (Table 3.42.2; see the clinical box). Tuberculosis is a very important cause of lung infection and is dealt with separately in Ch. 43. The clinical features of pneumonia include fever, general malaise and a productive cough. The inflammatory process not uncommonly spreads to the pleura (pleurisy) and this is associated with chest pain on inspiration.

Lobar pneumonia refers to pneumonia involving one pulmonary lobe, or part of a lobe, with infection spreading through the lobe via tiny holes in the alveolar walls (pores of Kohn; Fig. 3.42.1). This form of pneumonia may affect any age group

but most commonly affects young and middle-aged patients. **Bronchopneumonia** is a diffuse form of pneumonia that commonly involves both lungs (e.g. both lower lobes) and comprises inflammation centred on respiratory bronchioles. Bronchopneumonia is particularly common in elderly patients or those with an underlying serious disease (e.g. widespread cancer); in these patients, bronchopneumonia is a *very common* eventual cause of death.

Several factors may predispose to the development of pneumonia. The most common precipitating factors include severe underlying diseases, such as advanced cancer, and conditions in which the swallowing and/or cough reflex is impaired (e.g. stroke and degenerative brain diseases such as Alzheimer's disease). These conditions increase the risk of aspiration of gastric contents, which is the key event leading to the development of pneumonia. Malnutrition, diabetes mellitus and other conditions causing specific or generalized defects in the immune system (e.g. chemotherapy, HIV infection, congenital immunodeficiency states) will increase the risk of pneumonia as well as the risk of other infections.

Table 3.42.1 TYPES OF ORGANISM INFECTING THE LUNG

Organism	Features
Bacteria	Common; wide range of types (Table 3.42.2); usually severe and potentially life threatening
Viruses	Common but usually less severe than bacterial pneumonia
Fungi	Rare, e.g. *Pneumocystis carinii* pneumonia in HIV infection; *Aspergillus* sp. in immunocompromised patients

Table 3.42.2 BACTERIA CAUSING PNEUMONIA

Bacterial type	Characteristics
Gram positive	
Streptococcus pneumoniae	Common; CA; LP; BP; ECD
Staphylococcus aureus	Less common; HA; abscess-forming
Gram negative	
Haemophilus influenzae	Less common; CA; neonates; ECD
Enteric organisms e.g. *Escherischia coli*	Less common; severe; HA; BP; ECD
Legionella pneumophila	Legionnaire's disease; organism lives in tepid/stagnant water
Other	
Mycobacteria	Tuberculosis (Ch. 43.); atypical mycobacteria, e.g. in HIV infection
Mycoplasma pneumoniae[a]	Quite common; CA; less severe; radiograph changes worse than clinical signs
Chlamydia pneumoniae[a]	CA; less severe

CA, community acquired; HA, hospital acquired; LP, lobar pneumonia; BP, bronchopneumonia; ECD, exacerbation of chronic obstructive pulmonary disease.
[a]Mycoplasma and Chlamydia are important causes of 'atypical' pneumonias and are associated with an interstitial pneumonia pattern of inflammation.

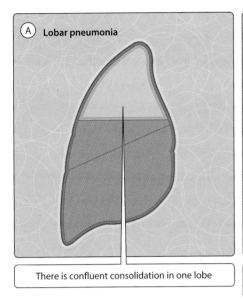
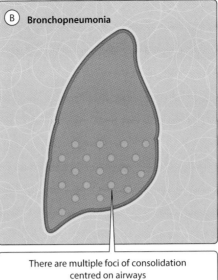

(A) Lobar pneumonia

There is confluent consolidation in one lobe

(B) Bronchopneumonia

There are multiple foci of consolidation centred on airways

Fig. 3.42.1 Pneumonia.

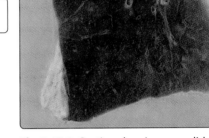

Fig. 3.42.2 Section showing consolidation in the upper lobe.

Clinical presentation

Clinical examination will reveal the signs of **consolidation** (i.e. inflammation within the lung leading to solidification of the lung tissue; Fig. 3.42.2):

- a dull percussion note
- bronchial breathing associated with crepitations on chest auscultation (stethoscope examination)
- a pleural rub heard via the stethoscope if pleurisy is present.

Radiological examination will reveal consolidation as shadowing, reflecting increased lung tissue density. These clinical and radiological features are more apparent in lobar pneumonia but will also be present in a more diffuse manner in bronchopneumonia.

PNEUMONIA IN HIV INFECTION

A 32-year-old homosexual man presented with a cough together with shortness of breath and general malaise. He admitted having multiple sexual partners over the last 8 years. Examination revealed clinical evidence of a chest infection. Initial investigations revealed a low total white cell count with CD4 cell count of less than 200×10^6 cells/l. A further blood test revealed the presence of antibodies to the HIV virus (i.e. that he was HIV positive). A chest radiograph revealed bilateral pulmonary shadowing, and cytopathological examination of a sputum sample revealed the presence of pneumocystic organisms. A diagnosis of *Pneumocystis carinii* (now known as *P. jirovecii*) pneumonia associated with AIDS was made and the patient was treated with antiretroviral therapy for the HIV infection together with co-trimoxazole antibiotic therapy for the pneumocystic infection. His respiratory symptoms resolved and his blood lymphocyte count returned to the normal range with this treatment.

Treatment

Bacterial pneumonia requires antibiotic therapy (commonly administered intravenously, especially with more severe forms of pneumonia) together with supportive treatment such as pain relief and inhaled oxygen. The inflammation can affect the pleura or pericardium and the infection can spread beyond the lungs.

Viral pneumonia affects the lung in a diffuse manner, characterized by chronic inflammation within alveolar walls (i.e. a form of interstitial pneumonia). Viral pneumonia tends to be less severe than bacterial pneumonia and will usually resolve spontaneously if supportive treatment is given; specific antiviral agents are not usually available.

Pneumonia often resolves fully with appropriate treatment and in these circumstances the lung tissue commonly returns entirely to normal. However, sometimes fibrosis (scarring) occurs and may affect the lung parenchyma (when severe, leading to interference with lung function) or the pleura (commonly occurring and resulting in pleural adhesions).

43. Tuberculosis

Questions
- Why is tuberculosis increasing in incidence?
- What are the clinical and pathological features of tuberculosis?

Tuberculosis is an extremely important cause of disease on a worldwide basis; although relatively uncommon in developed countries, it is currently increasing in incidence in the UK. This increase caused by several factors, including increased racial heterogeneity within the UK, altered living conditions within some sections of the population (e.g. living in overcrowded conditions) and an increased influx of people already infected with tuberculosis. The rise in incidence of HIV infection is also an important factor, not only within the UK but also particularly in zones where HIV infection is especially common (e.g. sub-Saharan Africa). Tuberculosis classically affects the lungs although it is a multisystem disease.

Causative organism

Tuberculosis is caused by mycobaterial infection, with classical tuberculosis associated with *Mycobacterium tuberculosis*. Other forms of mycobacteria exist and cause a range of related infections in a variety of clinical circumstances (Table 3.43.1). Mycobacteria are slender bacilli that are characteristically stained with the Ziehl–Neelsen stain based on their ability to retain a dye after acid and alcohol washes (acid- and alcohol-fast bacilli; AAFB). The bacteria cannot be cultured using conventional media and instead require special media such as the Lowenstein–Jensen medium, together with a prolonged incubation time of up to 6 weeks.

Pathological features

Macroscopic appearances

The hallmark lesion of tuberculosis is **caseous** (cheese-like, in reference to the marked tissue destruction associated with tuberculous infection and the featureless nature of the necrosis, in contrast to the more common coagulative necrosis in which

some elements of the tissue structure remain) with surrounding granulomatous inflammation. Foci of caseation appear macroscopically as soft pale areas between a few millimetres and several centimetres in size.

Microscopic appearances

Areas of caseation appear microscopically as foci of amorphous necrotic material surrounded by *granulomatous* inflammation in which multinucleate giant cells are found (Langhans' cells are also present; see Ch. 6). Ziehl–Neelsen staining reveals mycobacteria within macrophages or within the necrotic material in many, but not all, cases; consequently, a pathologist may not be able to exclude the possibility of mycobacterial infection if granulomatous inflammation is present, even if no mycobacteria are identified (Table 3.43.2). In these circumstances, identification of mycobaterial DNA using the polymerase chain reaction may allow confirmation of the diagnosis.

Patterns of infection

Figure 3.43.1 shows the patterns of infection that occur.

Primary infection

The classical primary infection is pulmonary and occurs in children, where it is characterized by a peripheral focus of infection (**Ghon focus**) together with enlarged pulmonary hilar lymph nodes (together forming a **Ghon complex**). This form of infection may be asymptomatic. Primary infection may also occur within the gastrointestinal tract in bovine tuberculosis, where the classical location is the ileocaecal region.

Reactivated infection

Following primary infection, mycobacteria commonly persist within the body, presumably within macrophages, where they may continue to exist for many years or even decades without causing clinical evidence of infection within immunocompetent individuals. However, subsequent immunocompromise can lead

Table 3.43.1   MYCOBACTERIAL INFECTIONS

Species	Disease
M. tuberculosis	Classical tuberculosis
M. bovis	Bovine tuberculosis
Atypical mycobacteria: M. avium intracellulare	Infections in immunocompromised patients
M. leprae	Leprosy
M. marinarum	Fish tank granuloma

Table 3.43.2   DISEASES CHARACTERIZED BY GRANULOMATOUS INFLAMMATION

Occurrence	Diseases
Common	Mycobacterial infections; Crohn's disease; sarcoidosis; reactions to foreign material
Unusual diseases	Fungal infections (some); *Yersinia* enterocolitis; *Campylobacter* enteritis; Wegener's granulomatosis

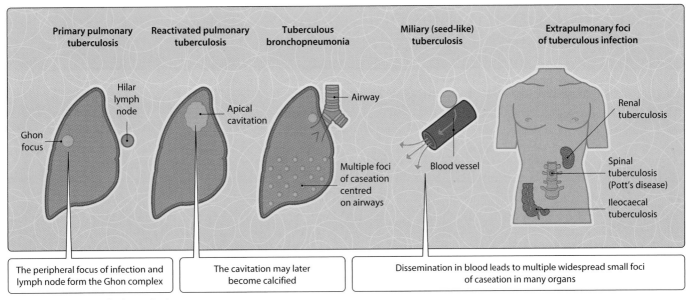

Fig. 3.43.1 Types of tuberculosis.

to proliferation of the bacteria with reemergence of infection (post primary tuberculosis). Factors that may lead to reactivated infection include:

- iatrogenic, e.g. chemotherapy, steroid therapy
- viral infection, e.g. HIV
- poor general health
- poor diet.

Reactivated pulmonary tuberculosis classically occurs within the lung apices because of their relatively well-oxygenated status. It results in severe damage to the lung tissue, with cavity formation and associated subsequent dystrophic calcification.

Tuberculous bronchopneumonia

Mycobacterial infection may extend into a bronchus and extend widely into the distal associated lung tissue in a bronchopneumonia pattern.

Miliary tuberculosis

Miliary (seed-like) tuberculosis most commonly occurs in immunocompromised individuals and results from blood-borne dissemination of infection with a widespread distribution. This results in very widespread small foci of caseation, resembling seeds, and is commonly fatal.

Other sites of infection

Ileocaecal tuberculosis results from the ingestion of unpasteurized milk and may produce clinical symptoms that are very similar to those of Crohn's disease. Both tuberculosis and Crohn's disease are characterized microscopically by the presence of granulomas, but intestinal tuberculosis tends to be associated with more florid granuloma formation and with the presence of caseous necrosis—a feature not seen in association with the granulomas of Crohn's disease.

Tuberculosis may occur within the kidney, where it results in haematuria and often with a palpable renal mass. Examination of early morning urine specimens for the presence of mycobacteria may help to confirm the diagnosis. Tuberculosis may involve the spine (**Pott's disease**) where the marked tissue destruction characterizing tuberculosis may result in collapse of vertebrae and pronounced spinal deformity. Other organs frequently involved include the adrenal glands, skin, lymph nodes, brain and epididymis.

44. Chronic obstructive pulmonary disease

Questions
- What is chronic obstructive pulmonary disease?
- What are its clinical and pathological features?

Chronic obstructive pulmonary disease (COPD) is a condition characterized by progressive lung damage associated with gradually worsening lung function. It has two main disease elements, **emphysema** and **chronic bronchitis**, which may be present alone or, more commonly, in combination. Cigarette smoking is by far the most common cause of COPD.

Emphysema

Emphysema is a process of lung parenchyma destruction in which the damage occurs distal to the respiratory bronchioles (i.e. tissue damage is centred on the alveolar walls). This process leads to the development of spaces of variable size within the lung parenchyma and to thin-walled sac-like structures over the surfaces of the lungs (**emphysematous bullae**; Fig. 3.44.1). Two patterns of alveolar wall destruction may occur. Smoking-related emphysema is characterized by centrilobular emphysema in which the damage is centred on respiratory bronchioles. Emphysema may also, much more rarely, occur in association with a genetically determined enzymatic defect (α_1-antitrypsin deficiency); this defect leads to **panacinar emphysema**, in which the damage is evenly distributed throughout the lung tissue.

Chronic bronchitis

Chronic bronchitis is defined clinically as a condition in which a productive cough is present for at least 3 months of the year and over at least 2 consecutive years. Marked thickening of bronchial walls characterizes the disease pathologically, mainly caused by the prominence of bronchial mucus glands (Fig. 3.44.1).

Clinical features

Both emphysema and chronic bronchitis cause *obstructive* lung defects and are, therefore, associated with poor lung function (Fig. 3.44.2). Emphysema reduces the normal elastic recoil within the lung parenchyma, which is the mechanism that preserves airway patency. Chronic bronchitis results in an obstructive defect through excess bronchial mucus production and fibrous scarring within bronchi. Emphysematous bullae may rupture, leading to the development of a pneumothorax. Patients with COPD are especially prone to recurrent lung infections, which further exacerbate poor lung function and which frequently require hospital-based treatment.

Patients with COPD usually have chronically low arterial oxygen saturations. Patients with predominant emphysema often also show a normal or low blood carbon dioxide concentration while those with predominant chronic bronchitis usually show a raised blood carbon dioxide concentration (carbon dioxide retention). The physiological trigger to breathe (respiratory drive) is usually provided by minute rises in blood carbon dioxide levels and this normal reflex is lost in patients who

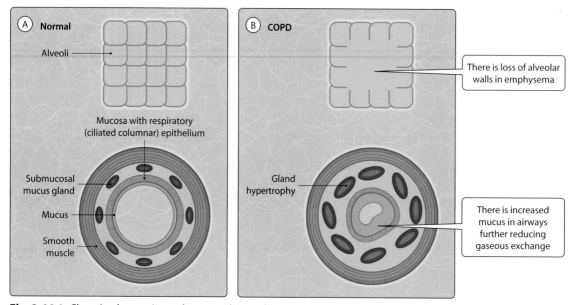

Fig. 3.44.1 Chronic obstructive pulmonary disease has progressive lung damage associated with two main disease elements: emphysema and chronic bronchitis. These usually both occur together.

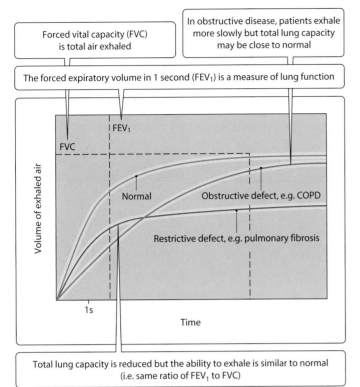

Forced vital capacity (FVC) is total air exhaled

In obstructive disease, patients exhale more slowly but total lung capacity may be close to normal

The forced expiratory volume in 1 second (FEV$_1$) is a measure of lung function

FEV$_1$

FVC

Volume of exhaled air

Normal

Obstructive defect, e.g. COPD

Restrictive defect, e.g. pulmonary fibrosis

1s

Time

Total lung capacity is reduced but the ability to exhale is similar to normal (i.e. same ratio of FEV$_1$ to FVC)

Fig. 3.44.2 Lung function tests. Spirometry tracings from three individuals: one normal, one with a restrictive lung disease and one with an obstructive lung disease (COPD). The subject is asked to blow into the spirometer as hard and as fast as possible. The volume expired in 6 seconds (FEV$_6$) is commonly used as a surrogate measure of forced vital capacity.

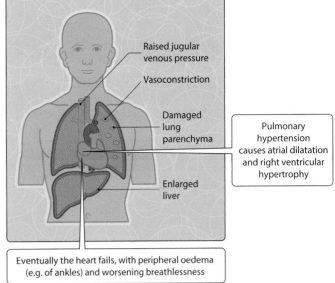

Raised jugular venous pressure

Vasoconstriction

Damaged lung parenchyma

Pulmonary hypertension causes atrial dilatation and right ventricular hypertrophy

Enlarged liver

Eventually the heart fails, with peripheral oedema (e.g. of ankles) and worsening breathlessness

Fig. 3.44.3 Cor pulmonale: heart failure secondary to chronic lung disease.

'retain' carbon dioxide. Respiratory drive is instead provided in these patients by a low blood oxygen level; if this is corrected via high-dose oxygen therapy then such patients lose their respiratory drive and can stop breathing. It is, therefore, important to *avoid the use of high-dose oxygen therapy* in patients with COPD whose blood carbon dioxide level is increased.

Cardiac failure

COPD results in poor alveolar ventilation and, therefore, a relatively low oxygen tension within alveoli. The pulmonary vasculature undergoes *vasoconstriction* in response to low oxygen

tension (unlike the systemic vasculature, which would undergo vasodilatation in these circumstances). This is a normal physiological mechanism that helps to divert blood to the best-ventilated areas of lung tissue, thereby optimizing gaseous exchange. However, in the presence of a severe global condition such as COPD, widespread pulmonary vasoconstriction occurs and this leads to increased pulmonary vascular resistance, pulmonary hypertension and increased strain on the right ventricle. Chronic increased right ventricular strain results in right ventricular hypertrophy and eventually in right ventricular cardiac failure. Right ventricular cardiac failure has characteristic clinical features (peripheral oedema, an engorged liver and a raised jugular venous pressure) and when occurring secondary to chronic lung disease is sometimes termed **cor pulmonale** (Fig. 3.44.3 and 3.40.1 D, p. 91).

45. Asthma

Question

- What is asthma?
- What are its clinical and pathological features?
- What are the four types of immune hypersensitivity?

The term asthma refers to a group of allergic conditions characterized by reversible pulmonary airway obstruction. Patients with the most common form of asthma commonly show genetic predisposition to related allergic conditions such as allergic dermatitis and hay fever, and these individuals are described as **atopic**.

Asthma and hay fever are the most well known of a spectrum of disorders caused by inappropriate immune activity (hypersensitivity).

Aetiology

Asthma may occur at any age but is most common among children and young adults. Several factors may precipitate an acute asthma attack and these are sometimes considered as either extrinsic or intrinsic:

- extrinsic
  – inhaled external antigens, e.g. dusts
- intrinsic
  – exercise
  – anxiety
  – cold air
  – infection, e.g. viral bronchitis.

While atopic asthma is the most common form of extrinsic asthma, other forms include occupational asthma and allergic bronchopulmonary aspergillosis; the latter is an IgE-mediated allergic reaction to *Aspergillus* colonization of the airways.

Clinical presentation

Breathlessness and wheezing are the dominant symptoms while examination may reveal an overexpanded chest and confirm the presence of wheezes on stethoscope examination (auscultation). Lung function testing reveals an *obstructive* pattern of defect (Fig. 3.44.2). Asthma attacks vary in severity, with severe attacks requiring hospital treatment. The most severe form of asthma attack is termed **status asthmaticus** and this can lead to respiratory failure and death unless prompt treatment is given.

Pathological features

Patients do not usually undergo lung biopsy for asthma so the pathological appearances are normally only seen at postmortem. The macroscopic features of the lungs in individuals dying from asthma are varied but classically show areas of parenchymal over-inflation and collapse together with widespread mucus plugging of airways. Microscopic examination additionally reveals eosinophilic infiltration and oedema within airway walls and loss of lining epithelium. Lungs from those who had long-standing disease may also show thickening of the epithelial basement

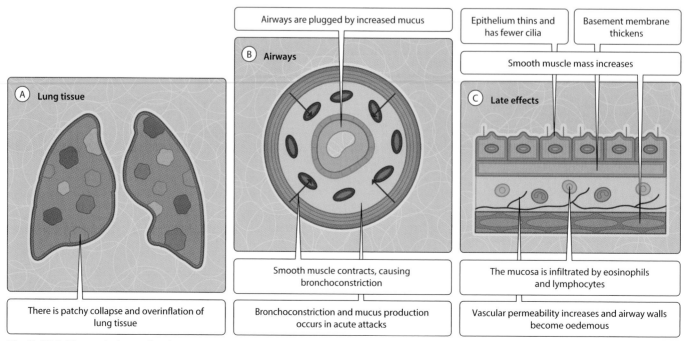

Fig. 3.45.1 The pathology of asthma.

membrane, with prominent mucus glands, smooth muscle proliferation and fibrosis within airway walls (Fig. 3.45.1).

Patients with asthma not uncommonly produce sputum samples that contain spirals of epithelium termed **Curschmann's spirals**; this may be a useful sign of asthma when identified during the cytological examination of sputum samples.

Immunopathology of asthma

The immunological mechanisms leading to asthma have been most precisely determined for extrinsic atopic asthma. In this condition, airways obstruction is caused by a type I (immediate) hypersensitivity reaction, leading to spasm of bronchial wall smooth muscle (resulting in bronchoconstriction), bronchial wall oedema and excess mucus production (resulting in plugging of airways). Therefore, extrinsic atopic asthma is an example of a Th1-mediated disease. Activated Th2 cells release cytokines (e.g. IL-4 and IL-5) that promote IgE synthesis and an increase in numbers of mast cells and eosinophils. The early phase of acute asthma (first 30 minutes) is mediated by cytokines, such as leukotrienes B_4, C_4, D_4 and E_4, together with prostaglandin D_2, platelet-activating factor and factors chemotactic for eosinophils and neutrophils. The late phase (several hours later) is mediated by cytokines such as TNF-α, which promotes recruitment of leukocytes; the leukocytes (especially eosinophils) further increase vascular permeability and cause epithelial cell damage. The reduction of nitric oxide concentrations resulting from epithelial cell damage may exacerbate bronchoconstriction.

Treatment

Most patients with asthma will become aware of the factors that trigger asthma attacks. Some of these factors may either be avoidable or predictable, for example a period of exercise. The mainstay of asthma treatment is inhaler therapy, most commonly with a β_2-agonist such as salbutamol, which relaxes bronchial smooth muscle and reduces mucus formation. Inhaled steroids may also reduce airway inflammation. Severe attacks resulting in hospitalization may need a combination of inhaled oxygen and nebulized β_2-agonist treatment while the most severe attacks may require ventilatory support.

Hypersensitivity

The term hypersensitivity is used to describe secondary damage to host tissue during the immune response to an antigen. Sometimes, the immune reaction and consequent tissue damage are out of all proportion to any risk posed by the antigen, for example when pollen causes hay fever or poison ivy causes a rash; the term 'allergy' is often used for such reactions.

Four main mechanisms are described and it can be useful to think of hypersensitivity reactions in terms of these four types.

Type I. This is the result of antigen binding to IgE on the surface of mast cells, which degranulate and thus initiate an inflammatory reaction. Type I reactions are important in hay fever, asthma and anaphylactic shock.

Type II. Antibodies bind to host tissues causing disease; this reaction is important in many autoimmune diseases, such as Goodpasture syndrome, in which antibody binds to the basement membrane of glomeruli and alveoli. Type II reactions also occur in transfusion reactions in which host antibodies recognize transfused blood cells as foreign.

Type III. Immune complexes are deposited in tissues. Immune complexes are aggregates of antibody and antigen that form in certain circumstances; they can be deposited locally or at a distant site, typically in blood vessel walls. This process is important in many rheumatological diseases (e.g. systemic lupus erythematosus).

Type IV. Whereas types I–III reactions are mediated by antibodies, type IV hypersensitivity is caused by antibody binding to T cells. This process is important in the host response to many microorganisms that live inside cells (e.g. mycobacteria), because the activated T cells induce apoptosis in infected cells. It also occurs in organ transplant rejection and in certain allergies (e.g. poison ivy rash).

46. Restrictive lung diseases

Questions
- What is restrictive lung disease?
- What are the main causes of restrictive lung disease?

The defining feature of restrictive lung diseases is reduced compliance (i.e. increased stiffness) of the lungs, thoracic cage or both. The basic defect can be seen on a spirometer tracing (Fig. 3.44.2). Patients with restrictive lung diseases cannot fill their lungs normally, and so the total amount of air they have in their lungs is reduced and the forced vital capacity (FVC), which is the total amount of air that is expelled from the lungs by forced expiration after a full inspiration, is low. However, there is no obstruction to outflow, so they can blow out the air quickly and the forced expiratory volume in one second (FEV_1) is in proportion to their lung volume. Therefore, the FEV_1:FVC ratio is approximately normal. In contrast, patients with obstructive lung disease (Ch. 44) have normal (or even enlarged) lung volumes, but they cannot blow the air out quickly because of the airway obstruction. Therefore, their FEV_1:FVC ratio is reduced.

The main causes of restrictive lung disease can be classified according to whether they involve the lungs themselves (pulmonary causes) or structures outside the lungs (extrapulmonary causes) (Fig. 3.46.1).

Pulmonary causes

Acute respiratory distress syndrome

Acute respiratory distress syndrome (ARDS) is caused by an acute injury to the walls of the alveoli and respiratory bronchioles. The pathogenesis can be divided into two major types depending on the aetiology of the lung injury.

Type 1, inflammatory. Acute inflammation of the alveoli and respiratory bronchioles is the primary abnormality; aetiologies include pneumonia, aspiration of gastric contents, septicaemia, shock, pulmonary contusion, fat embolism and inhalation of irritants such as toxic fumes. The type II pneumocytes (producing surfactant, whereas type I are involved in gas exchange) are damaged as part of this process and consequently there is a secondary failure of surfactant production, resulting in alveolar collapse.

Type 2, failure of surfactant production in premature infants. Here, failure of surfactant production by the type II pneumocytes of the immature lungs is the *primary* defect. The lack of surfactant causes alveolar collapse, which causes hypoxia. As a consequence of hypoxia, pulmonary vasoconstriction

occurs, and the pulmonary hypoperfusion causes secondary damage to alveolar walls.

Both types of acute lung injury cause fluid and blood to leak into the alveoli, causing pulmonary oedema, and damage the pneumocytes, which become necrotic. The alveolar ducts and alveoli become lined by a **hyaline membrane** composed of fibrinous inflammatory exudate and necrotic epithelial cells. This hyaline membrane is a characteristic feature of ARDS. Indeed, a previous name for ARDS, especially in premature infants, was hyaline membrane disease. The lack of surfactant, whether in prematurity or secondary to damage to type II pneumocytes, causes alveolar collapse, and patches of lung in which the air spaces are not expanded appear. The name given to these areas of collapsed, uninflated lung is **atelectasis**.

After about a week, the process enters a reparative phase. Neutrophils disappear, and macrophages dispose of hyaline membranes by phagocytosis. There is proliferation of type II pneumocytes, which ultimately differentiate into type I pneumocytes, restoring the normal alveolar epithelium. Proliferation and activation of interstitial fibroblasts produces interstitial fibrosis (i.e. collagenous thickening of alveolar walls). If the alveolar walls are only mildly thickened, the patient may recover with essentially normal lung function. However, more marked fibrosis can result in distortion of lung parenchyma and reduced gas exchange.

Chronic interstitial lung diseases

The chronic interstitial lung diseases have a number of common features. They are characterized pathologically by interstitial fibrosis caused by scarring of the walls of the airways, and clinically produce restrictive lung defects. In the later stages, the lung may show a change known as **honeycomb lung**, in which dilated air spaces lined by type II pneumocytes are surrounded by fibrotic tissue. Examples of interstitial lung disease include idiopathic pulmonary fibrosis (cryptogenic fibrosing alveolitis), pneumoconioses, sarcoidosis, hypersensitivity pneumonitis, connective tissue diseases (e.g. systemic lupus erythematosus), and drug-associated pulmonary fibrosis. Some of these conditions are discussed.

Pneumoconioses

Pneumoconiosis describes a fibrotic lung reaction to inhaled dusts. By definition, it excludes both the allergic alveolitides, which are hypersensitivity reactions, and also neoplasms caused by inhaled dusts. In general, the dusts causing pneumoconiosis are inorganic, whereas organic material induces allergic alveolitis.

Examples of dusts that cause interstitial lung disease are coal dust (coal-workers' pneumoconiosis), asbestos (asbestosis) and silica (silicosis).

Common to all pneumoconioses is the deposition of dust in the lung, where it is taken up by alveolar macrophages. Exactly where and how much dust is deposited depends on the size and shape of the particles, the airflow through the lungs and the efficiency with which particles are trapped in the respiratory mucus. Large particles are readily trapped in the mucus layer and disposed of; very small particles tend to move in and out of the alveoli without being deposited. However, particles 1–5 µm in diameter tend to be deposited at the bifurcations of alveolar ducts. These dust particles are taken up by macrophages, which may then secrete pro-inflammatory cytokines and release free radicals that directly damage tissue. In general, the risk of developing pneumoconiosis increases with the amount of exposure to the dust. In addition, tobacco smoking potentiates the effect of mineral dusts, an effect that is particularly notable with asbestosis.

Sarcoidosis

Sarcoidosis is a multisystem disease characterized by granulomatous inflammation. The clinical manifestations are highly variable, since any organ system can be affected, but it is convenient to consider the disease here because one of its commonest manifestations is lung involvement with dyspnoea, cough, chest pain and a restrictive lung defect.

The aetiology is unknown, although some evidence points to an environmental or infectious cause. It seems that processing of an antigen (as yet unidentified) by macrophages triggers an oligoclonal expansion of CD4 T-cells of the Th1 subtype, resulting in increased levels of Th1 cytokines. The initial response is amplified, and macrophages and T-cells aggregate to form granulomas. These granulomas are composed of epithelioid macrophages and multinucleated giant cells surrounded by a zone of T-cells are characteristic of sarcoidosis. Caseation, which would be suggestive of tuberculosis, is not observed. The inflammation may resolve or fibrosis may follow.

The outcome varies from spontaneous resolution and complete recovery to progressive disease with organ failure. Approximately 5% of patients die as result.

Allergic alveolitis (hypersensitivity pneumonitis)

Allergic alveolitis is an immunogically mediated lung disease. Allergens include fungi in mouldy hay (farmer's lung), thermophilic actinomycetes in cool-mist humidifiers (humidifier lung) and pigeon droppings (pigeon-fancier's lung). Type III and type IV hypersensitivity reactions appear to be involved.

The inflammation affects the alveoli, causing chronic inflammation that is usually granulomatous. There is diffuse interstitial fibrosis in long-standing disease.

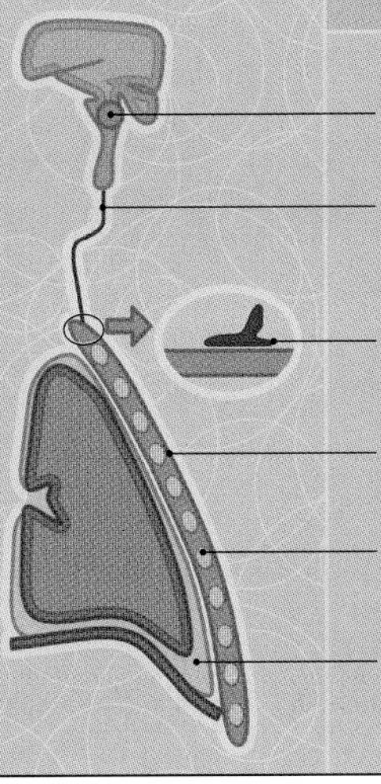

	Site	Pathophysiology	Examples
	Respiratory centres in brain	Reduced central respiratory drive	Cerebral trauma, drugs (e.g. opiates)
	Nerves	Interruption of nerve supply to respiratory muscle	Polio, Guillain–Barré syndrome
	Neuromuscular junctions	Reduced neuromuscular transmission	Myasthenia gravis
	Respiratory muscles	Muscular weakness	Muscular dystrophy
	Thoracic cage	Deformity or limitation of movement	Kyphoscoliosis, severe obesity
	Pleural cavities	Reduced volume within pleural cavities	Pleural effusion, pneumothorax

Fig. 3.46.1 Extrapulmonary causes of restrictive lung defects.

47. Gastritis and peptic ulcer disease

Questions
- What is peptic ulceration and what are its main causes?
- How may it present clinically and what are its complications?

Peptic ulceration is defined as a breach in the mucosa (i.e. full-thickness loss) of the gastrointestinal tract caused by the action of acidic gastric juice. Peptic ulcers can be acute or chronic, although sometimes the term peptic ulcer is confined to the chronic variety (Fig. 3.47.1). Some types of inflammation of the stomach (gastritis) are especially associated with peptic ulcer formation, and these are discussed in this chapter.

Gastritis
Acute gastritis
The principal causes of acute gastritis are:
- **NSAIDs:** cause reduced prostaglandin synthesis in the gastric mucosa, leading to exfoliation of surface epithelial cells and inhibition of mucus secretion, thus reducing mucosal defences against acid attack
- **alcohol** (ethanol): direct irritant of the lining of the stomach
- **stress** (e.g. severe burns, major trauma): associated with gastric inflammation, erosion and ulceration, possibly as a result of mucosal ischaemia
- **bile reflux:** reflux of bile through the pylorus from the duodenum.

Acute gastritis is often associated with partial-thickness defects in the mucosa. Such defects are sometimes called **erosions** (as opposed to an ulcer, which is a full-thickness breach). These erosions often bleed and may present as gastric haemorrhage. In severe cases, the erosions deepen to become true ulcers.

Chronic gastritis
Chronic gastritis can be generated by any of the causes of acute gastritis if they act for long enough. In addition, chronic gastritis can occur de novo through autoimmune mechanisms. For example, pernicious anaemia is an autoimmune condition in which damage to parietal cells causes loss of intrinsic factor and hence failure of vitamin B_{12} absorption. It is associated with inflammation and subsequent atrophy of the mucosa in the gastric body and fundus. However, the most common cause of chronic gastritis is infection with *Helicobacter pylori*.

Although *H. pylori* does not invade the tissues, it lives in the surface mucus of gastric mucosa (Fig. 3.47.2) where it secretes a number of toxins that damage surface epithelial cells and break down the mucus barrier. When first acquired, this organism produces a transient acute gastritis, but this is self-limiting and often produces no symptoms. Some individuals mount an effective defence and eliminate the organism. Many individuals do not clear the organism, however, and a chronic carrier state develops. This carrier state is associated with chronic inflammation of the mucosa driven by a Th1 immune response, the severity of the inflammation depending on the strain of the infecting organism. As a result, patients may either have abdominal symptoms or be asymptomatic. The most common serious sequela of *H. pylori* infection is peptic ulceration.

Peptic ulcers
Most peptic ulcers occur in the first portion of the duodenum, and most of the remainder occur in the stomach. Within the stomach, the typical site is at the junction between body and fundus mucosa on the lesser curve. Occasionally, peptic ulcers arise in the distal oesophagus, in Meckel diverticula and at gastroenterostomy sites.

Morphology
Chronic peptic ulcers have clear-cut margins, in contrast to the irregular, infiltrative margin of an ulcerated carcinoma. The base of a chronic peptic ulcer consists of necrotic slough and inflammatory exudate overlying granulation tissue. The latter is surrounded by a zone of fibrous scar tissue (Fig. 3.47.1). The whole lesion is infiltrated by inflammatory cells.

A deep ulcer can penetrate all the way through the muscularis propria into the perigastric adipose tissue. Arteries near the ulcer often show **endarteritis obliterans**, in which the lumen of

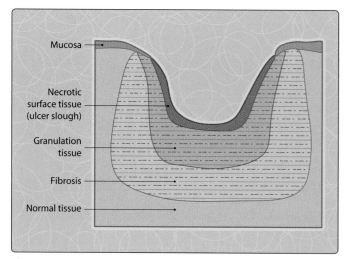

Fig. 3.47.1 Cross-section through a chronic peptic ulcer.

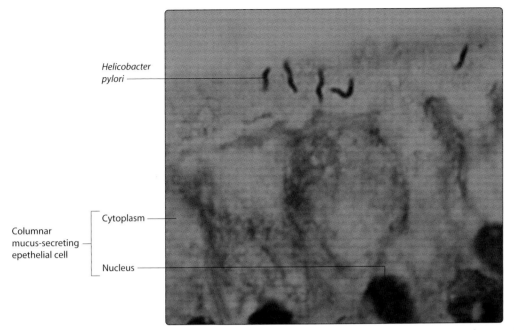

Helicobacter pylori

Cytoplasm

Columnar mucus-secreting epethelial cell

Nucleus

Fig. 3.47.2 *Helicobacter pylori* in the surface mucus of the stomach. Modified Giemsa stain, oil immersion lens.

the artery is markedly narrowed by intimal proliferation; this adaptive response can prevent massive haemorrhage if the artery is breached by the ulcerative process.

Pathogenesis

Gastric juice is a highly irritant cocktail including hydrochloric acid and pepsin. The principal line of defence of mucosal surfaces that come into contact with it is the mucus layer secreted by the mucosal epithelial cells. The effectiveness of the mucus layer is enhanced by bicarbonate ions within it, which have a buffering effect.

Most peptic ulceration results from reduced mucosal defences, in particular reduction in the mucus barrier or damage to the epithelial cells that secrete it. The main causes, which can act alone or in combination, are:

- *Helicobacter pylori*: occurs in association with chronic peptic ulcer in approximately 70% of patients with a stomach ulcer and 90% of patients with a duodenal ulcer; in the latter, it is thought that gastric metaplasia in the proximal duodenum is a site for colonization by *H. pylori*, which thus induces inflammation in the duodenum
- **NSAIDs**: inhibit prostaglandin synthesis, leading to reduced production of mucin and bicarbonate
- **cigarette smoking**: reduces mucosal blood flow; healing of injured mucosa is also impaired
- **corticosteroids**: steroid therapy is associated with an increased risk of peptic ulcer
- **psychological factors**: epidemiological evidence suggests that psychological stress may predispose to ulcer formation.

On rare occasions, the cause is not poor mucosal defences but enhanced acid attack. This is seen in Zollinger–Ellison syndrome: gastric hyperacidity caused by a gastrin-secreting tumour (usually a carcinoid tumour of the upper gastrointestinal tract).

H. pylori infection is also associated with increased risk of certain neoplasms. Many of those with chronic *H. pylori* gastritis exhibit intestinal metaplasia of the gastric mucosa. This is a risk factor for the development of gastric carcinoma: many gastric carcinomas arise from dysplasia developing in intestinal metaplasia. There is also an increased risk of B-cell lymphoma in *H. pylori* gastritis, and activation of B-cells as part of the immune response may represent the mechanism for lymphoma development in these cases.

Clinical presentation

Peptic ulcers typically cause pain, but other symptoms such as weight loss, nausea and vomiting may occur. Sometimes, peptic ulcers present with a complication, such as:

- perforation, with leakage of gastric contents into the peritoneal cavity and peritonitis
- penetration, in which an ulcer erodes into an adjacent organ (e.g. duodenal ulcer eroding into the pancreas)
- bleeding, from eroded vessels in the ulcer base, which can result in
  - iron-deficiency anaemia
  - massive haemorrhage with shock
  - melaena
  - haematemesis
- pyloric stenosis owing to scarring.

48. Malabsorption

Questions
- What are the clinical features of malabsorption?
- What are the most common causes of malabsorption?
- Why does coeliac disease occur?

Digestion involves enzymatic breakdown of proteins, carbohydrates and fats, and transport of nutrients across the intestinal epithelium into capillaries and lymphatics. Malabsorption implies a failure of these functions despite adequate nutritional intake. The most common causes in industrialized countries are pancreatic insufficiency, coeliac disease and Crohn disease (Fig. 3.48.1).

Clinical features of malabsorption

Steatorrhoea is the passage of stools containing undigested fat. They are pale and bulky with an offensive smell, float on water and are difficult to flush away. Steatorrhoea is found when there is:

- failure of fat breakdown within the gut lumen (e.g. pancreatic enzyme deficiency in pancreatic disease) or failure of solubilization of fat through lack of bile salts in biliary insufficiency
- inadequate fat absorption, caused by decreased absorptive surface area, microorganisms or lymphatic obstruction.

Osmotic diarrhoea results if there are undigested nutrients that cause large amounts of water to be retained in the stools by oncotic pressure. It can be found in any form of malabsorption but particularly in disaccharidase deficiency. Osmotic diarrhoea is watery, unless undigested fats turn it into steatorrhoea.

Weight loss is common and may be the presenting feature of a malabsorption syndrome. In infants and children, **failure to thrive** is a common finding.

Deficiency of fat-soluble vitamins can occur where there is a significant failure of fat absorption. Vitamin D deficiency can lead to hypocalcaemia, osteomalacia and rickets, while lack of vitamin K can result in hypoprothrombinaemia and a bleeding tendency. Lack of vitamin A is a theoretical possibility but in practice it is rarely observed in malabsorption syndromes.

Potassium depletion causes thirst, polyuria, paraesthesiae and muscle weakness, while **protein deficiency** can cause muscle wasting, hypoproteinaemia and oedema. **Anaemia** is a common feature of malabsorption and may be caused by failure to absorb iron, folate and/or vitamin B_{12}.

There may also be a variety of non-specific symptoms such as anorexia, abdominal distension, colicky pains, audible intestinal sounds (borborygmi) and excess flatus.

Coeliac disease

Coeliac disease (gluten-sensitive enteropathy) is an inflammatory disease of the small intestine caused by an abnormal immunological reaction to gluten (in wheat and other grains). Gluten is a complex substance that includes the protein gliadin. In susceptible individuals, peptides derived from gliadin stimulate an immune response in which lymphocytes and

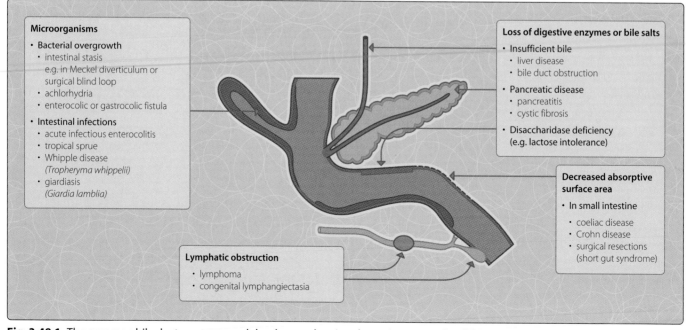

Fig. 3.48.1 The common bile duct, pancreas and duodenum showing the main causes of malabsorption.

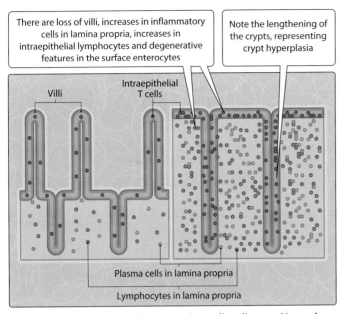

There are loss of villi, increases in inflammatory cells in lamina propria, increases in intraepithelial lymphocytes and degenerative features in the surface enterocytes

Note the lengthening of the crypts, representing crypt hyperplasia

Villi

Intraepithelial T cells

Plasma cells in lamina propria

Lymphocytes in lamina propria

Fig. 3.48.2 Morphological changes in coeliac disease. Normal small intestinal mucosa is shown on the left and that in coeliac disease on the right.

plasma cells sensitized to gliadin peptides infiltrate the lamina propria. It is this immune response that is responsible for the manifestations of the disease. Threfore, the treatment of coeliac disease is withdrawal of gluten from the diet. It takes some diligence on the part of individuals to keep to a gluten-free diet, since wheat flour is present in so many foods.

The prevalence of gluten intolerance depends on the diagnostic criteria used, but in European populations it is approximately 1 in 300 in a number of studies. The disease typically presents in children or young adults, but it can appear occasionally in older adults or the elderly. In some cases, iron-deficiency anaemia is the presenting feature, and for this reason tests for coeliac disease are indicated in patients with unexplained anaemia.

Diagnosis

Coeliac disease can be diagnosed by the characteristic morphological changes on small intestinal biopsy (Fig. 3.48.2). In the past, jejunal biopsy was the rule, but nowadays the usual specimen is a distal duodenal biopsy taken through a flexible endoscope. An increase in plasma cells and lymphocytes in lamina propria, and an increase in the numbers of intraepithelial T-cells is seen. There is crypt hyperplasia owing to increased proliferation of the stem cells in the crypts. At the same time, the villi flatten (villous atrophy). The surface enterocytes exhibit degenerative features. These changes are usually most pronounced in the proximal small intestine (duodenum and jejunum).

Serology can be useful in diagnosis. Patients are often positive for anti-tissue transglutaminase (anti-tTG), anti-gliadin and anti-endomysial antibodies. Anti-tTG is the most sensitive and specific test. In practice, the diagnosis usually rests on a combination of clinical features, biopsy and serology.

Complications

Patients with coeliac disease are at increased risk of malignant lymphoma. Although most lymphomas arising in the intestines are of B-cell type, in patients with coeliac disease the lymphomas tend to be of T-cell type. Coeliac disease is also associated with an increased incidence of carcinomas of the gastrointestinal tract.

Microbial causes of malabsorption

Many intestinal infections can disrupt digestive functions. One of them is **Whipple disease**, which is a rare infection caused by *Tropheryma whippelii*. It can affect any organ but most often involves the intestine, joints and central nervous system. Biopsies of the intestine show the lamina propria to be filled with granular macrophages containing the bacterium.

Tropical sprue is encountered in individuals who live in or have visited tropical or subtropical countries. It closely resembles gluten-sensitive enteropathy but does not involve gluten sensitivity. The precise cause is unclear, but it is believed to be a type of infectious enterocolitis. It responds to antibiotics.

Bacterial overgrowth can occur under certain circumstances. In health, the proximal small intestine contains moderate numbers of bacteria, although usually many orders of magnitude lower than in the large bowel. However, the concentration of bacteria in the small bowel can increase if there is stasis in a blind loop or diverticulum, achlorhydria (i.e. the stomach does not produce acid that would otherwise inhibit bacterial growth) or a fistula connecting the colon with the stomach or small bowel, allowing large intestinal bacteria direct access to the proximal gut. The mechanism whereby bacterial overgrowth causes malabsorption is obscure but it might involve modification of ingested nutrients by the bacteria, damage to brush borders of the intestinal cells and/or hydrolysis of bile salts.

Disaccharidase deficiency

The most common disaccharidase deficiency is of **lactase**, where patients experience symptoms after consuming lactose-rich foods such as milk. The commonest cause is a genetically inherited decrease in lactase activity with age, which typically becomes apparent between the ages of 5 and 20 years. Secondary lactase deficiency can be a feature of damage to the intestinal epithelium (where the lactase is found) caused by gastroenteritis, coeliac disease, inflammatory bowel disease and other related conditions.

49. Gallstones

Questions
- Why do gallstones occur?
- What are the complications of gallstone disease?

The condition of having gallstones is called **cholelithiasis**. It is common, particularly in industrialized countries, where postmortem studies have found an overall prevalence in adults of approximately 10–20% in the elderly. Females are affected two or three times more often as males. Gallstones are often asymptomatic but can cause inflammation or obstruction.

Stones (**calculi**) can form in other bodily fluids too (e.g. urine and saliva, causing urolithiasis and sialolithiasis, respectively). Some of the principles of stone formation described in this chapter, such as supersaturation and nucleation, apply to all of these sites.

Most gallstones consist of a mixture of bile pigments and cholesterol. Nevertheless, one of these constituents usually predominates, and so gallstones can be classified as being cholesterol stones or pigment stones. The significance of this classification stems from the different pathogenesis of the two types.

Pathogenesis

Cholesterol stones account for the majority of gallstones in industrialized countries, whereas they are uncommon in non-industrialized countries. The pathophysiology of their formation is summarized in Fig. 3.49.1. Cholesterol dissolves in bile through the detergent actions of lecithin and bile salts. If there is an excess of cholesterol, the solution becomes supersaturated and crystals of cholesterol monohydrate may precipitate *if* there is a nucleus on which they can begin to grow. Anything that acts as a substrate for crystal growth can act as a nucleus, for example a tiny crystal that forms spontaneously or a particle of mucus. The bile normally contains proteins that tend to inhibit nucleation (antinucleating proteins) and protect against the risk of crystal formation if the bile becomes supersaturated.

Two factors promote nucleation in a supersaturated solution. First, hypomotility of the gallbladder, with consequent biliary stasis, allows time for nucleation and crystal growth to occur. As high cholesterol concentration in bile inhibits gallbladder motility, the presence of a supersaturated solution will itself produce this effect. Second, the ratio of antinucleating proteins to pronucleating proteins falls (the mechanism of this process is unclear). Consequently, there is an increased tendency for small crystals to form and then grow into stones.

Morphologically, cholesterol stones are yellow and their crystalline structure is revealed on examination of a cut surface (Fig. 3.49.2). They tend to be hard and can grow to several centimetres in diameter. Pure cholesterol stones are unusual; most of them also contain some bilirubin and calcium salts. Cholesterol stones with a high proportion of other ingredients are sometimes called mixed stones. In approximately 10% of patients, they contain sufficient calcium to make them radio-opaque to X-rays. Whether calcified or not, gallstones are detectable by ultrasound.

Biliary sludge describes a mixture of cholesterol monohydrate crystals, mucus and calcium bilirubinate granules. It is believed to be the precursor of most gallstones and can be associated with biliary colic, acute cholecystitis and pancreatitis.

Pigment stones

Most gallbladder calculi in non-industrialized countries are pigment type. Formation of pigment stones is caused by increased levels of unconjugated bilirubin in the bile. Unconjugated bilirubin is poorly soluble in aqueous solution and readily precipitates as bilirubin salts, principally calcium bilirubinate. Pigment stones are brown or black, tend to be soft or crumbly, and rarely grow to more than 1.5 cm diameter. They may contain

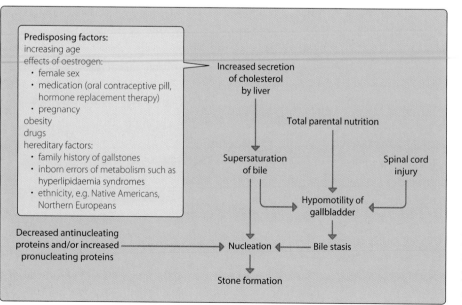

Fig. 3.49.1 Summary of the main pathways involved in the pathogenesis of cholesterol stones.

Predisposing factors:
increasing age
effects of oestrogen:
- female sex
- medication (oral contraceptive pill, hormone replacement therapy)
- pregnancy
obesity
drugs
hereditary factors:
- family history of gallstones
- inborn errors of metabolism such as hyperlipidaemia syndromes
- ethnicity, e.g. Native Americans, Northern Europeans

Decreased antinucleating proteins and/or increased pronucleating proteins

Increased secretion of cholesterol by liver

Total parental nutrition

Supersaturation of bile

Spinal cord injury

Hypomotility of gallbladder

Nucleation ← Bile stasis

Stone formation

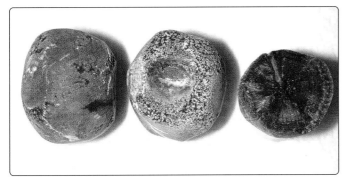

Fig. 3.49.2 Cholesterol gallstones. Calcium salts impart a greyish appearance. The stone on the right has been bisected and the cut surface reveals radiating crystals of yellow cholesterol monohydrate.

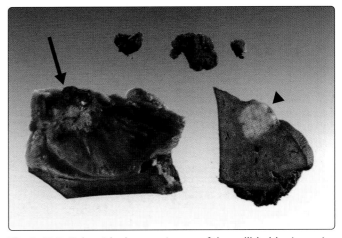

Fig. 3.49.3 Polypoid adenocarcinoma of the gallbladder (arrow) with liver metastasis (arrowhead). There were several mixed cholesterol calculi in the gallbladder, three of which are shown at the top of the image.

inorganic calcium salts and cholesterol monohydrate crystals. Many are radio-opaque. There are two main circumstances in which unconjugated bilirubin in the bile increases.

Haemolytic anaemia. Increased haemolysis increases the rate of production of bilirubin from haem. Consequently, the liver secretes a raised amount of conjugated bilirubin, but a fixed proportion (approximately 1%) becomes deconjugated in the biliary tree. Therefore, the concentration of unconjugated bilirubin may exceed its solubility and bilirubin salts will precipitate out of solution.

Biliary tract infections. Deconjugation of bilirubin glucuronides by hydrolysis is accelerated by bacteria or parasites such as liver flukes.

Clinical features and complications

Most patients with gallstones have no symptoms. However, there are many ways in which cholelithiasis can manifest clinically.

Biliary colic. If the gallbladder or biliary tree contracts spasmodically against the resistance of a gallstone, pain results.

Acute cholecystitis. Gallstones are the most common cause of acute cholecystitis. (Occasionally, acute cholecystitis occurs in the absence of gallstones. This condition is known as **acute acalculous cholecystitis** and usually follows severe trauma, extensive burns or major surgery.) In many cases, an obstructing stone at the neck of the gallbladder appears to precipitate an attack of acute cholecystitis. The gallbladder exhibits the usual features of acute inflammation described in more detail elsewhere in this book: the serosal surfaces show a fibrinous or fibrinopurulent exudate; the wall becomes congested, oedematous and infiltrated with neutrophils, sometimes with abscess formation; and the mucosa becomes ulcerated. If there is widespread necrosis of the wall, gangrenous cholecystitis may follow. If the lumen of the gallbladder becomes filled with pus, the term **empyema** of the gallbladder is used. If the inflammation subsides but the neck of the gallbladder remains blocked, the gallbladder lumen becomes filled with bile-free clear mucoid fluid (mucocoele of the gallbladder).

Perforation. Perforation is likely in gangrenous cholecystitis as there is weakening of the gallbladder wall.

Chronic cholecystitis. This is characterized by the presence of cells of chronic inflammation and thickening of the gallbladder wall by fibrosis. Outpouchings of the mucosa called **Rokitansky–Aschoff sinuses** are common and appear to be diverticula caused by intraluminal pressure pushing the mucosa through weakened areas of gallbladder wall.

Cholangitis. Stasis of bile predisposes to infection. The pathogens are usually enteric bacteria that cause an ascending infection of the biliary tree.

Obstructive jaundice. So long as the stones are confined to the gallbladder, bile can still pass from the liver into the duodenum and jaundice does not occur. However, if a stone enters the common bile duct, becomes impacted and blocks the flow of bile, obstructive jaundice results.

Pancreatitis. Gallstones are associated with an increased risk of pancreatitis.

Fistula. Occasionally, inflammation of the gallbladder wall is associated with the formation of a fistula to an adjacent hollow viscus or, rarely, the skin. If the fistulous tract leads to the small intestine and a gallstone passes through it, the gallstone, if it is large enough, can obstruct the intestine, causing a condition known as **gallstone ileus**.

Carcinoma. This appears to be more common in gallbladders with chronic inflammation, whether caused by stones (Fig. 3.49.3) or parasites. Most are adenocarcinomas. They have usually spread widely before they are discovered and the prognosis is poor.

50. Pancreatitis

Questions
- Why does pancreatitis occur?
- What are the complications of pancreatitis?
- What is the difference between acute and chronic pancreatitis?

Inflammation of the pancreas may be acute or chronic. Acute pancreatitis implies the sudden onset of inflammation with, in severe cases, haemorrhagic necrosis. In chronic pancreatitis, the inflammation causes fibrosis and atrophy of acinar tissue with irreversible impairment of pancreatic function.

Acute pancreatitis

Aetiology and pathogenesis

There are a number of causes of acute pancreatitis;

- toxins: ethanol, drugs (e.g. diuretics such as thiazides and furosemide), venoms (e.g. certain scorpion stings)
- obstruction of the pancreatic ducts: gallstones, tumours of the ampulla of Vater, parasites (e.g. ascariasis and liver flukes)
- infections: mumps, coxsackievirus
- metabolic disorders: hypercalcaemia, hypothermia, hyperlipidaemia
- mechanical injury: trauma, endoscopic procedures involving cannulation or injection of the pancreatic ducts
- ischaemia: shock, obstruction of blood supply (e.g. arterial embolism)
- genetic: inherited abnormalities in genes encoding pancreatic enzymes and their inhibitors.

The commonest causes in industrialized countries are gallstones and alcohol abuse, which together account for approximately three-quarters of all cases. There is no known cause in approximately 10%.

The pathogenesis of acute pancreatitis is poorly understood. Recent research has suggested that toxic damage promotes free radical production together with activation of mast cells. It is also believed that autodigestion of the pancreatic tissue by pancreatic enzymes is involved. Normally, pancreatic enzymes do not attack the pancreatic tissues because:

- the enzymes are physically isolated from other cellular components within the endoplasmic reticulum, Golgi apparatus and secretory granules
- many enzymes are stored as inactive precursors
- enzyme inhibitors (e.g. serine protease inhibitor) protect the pancreas from any active enzyme inadvertently released.

In acute pancreatitis, activation of digestive enzymes, for example phospholipase and elastase, and their release into the cell and surrounding tissues promote the haemorrhagic necrosis characteristic of severe pancreatitis. Amylase and lipase are released into the bloodstream, and raised serum amylase and lipase are used as diagnostic tests for acute pancreatitis.

The relationship between gallstones and acute pancreatitis is unclear. It is often assumed that gallstones act by obstructing the outflow of pancreatic juice if they impact at the ampulla of Vater. However, only a minority of patients with gallstones complicated by acute pancreatitis have a demonstrable stone obstructing the ampulla.

Pathology

In mild pancreatitis, the pancreas is swollen and oedematous. In more severe cases, necrosis of the pancreatic parenchyma occurs; there is typically extensive haemorrhage because of destruction of vessel walls (possibly by released proteases) and the appearance is described as **acute haemorrhagic pancreatitis**. In the most severe instances, the pancreas is transformed into a necrotic haemorrhagic mass in which pancreatic tissue is barely recognizable. The inflammation causes pain, and the commonest presenting feature is continuous epigastric pain, which often radiates to the back.

Fat necrosis from the action of lipase released from the damaged pancreas is common in the surrounding tissues. It is characterized by saponification (the chemical production of soaps) and calcium deposition, and the necrotic fat takes on a soft chalky appearance. The sequestration of calcium in the necrotic fat can cause hypocalcaemia. Occasionally, circulating lipase can cause subcutaneous fat necrosis in the lower limbs and elsewhere.

Patients may become hypotensive, with shock caused by the release into the circulation of inflammatory mediators (e.g. cytokines and bradykinin). Severe shock can cause death by multiorgan failure.

Many patients who recover develop **pancreatic pseudocysts**, which are spaces lined by connective tissue containing necrotic debris and blood. They are not true cysts because they are not lined by epithelium. Pseudocysts may become secondarily infected and form an abscess. Large ones can press on adjacent structures.

Chronic pancreatitis

Aetiology and pathogenesis

Many of the causes of acute pancreatitis can lead to chronic pancreatitis. The main aetiological factors are as follows.

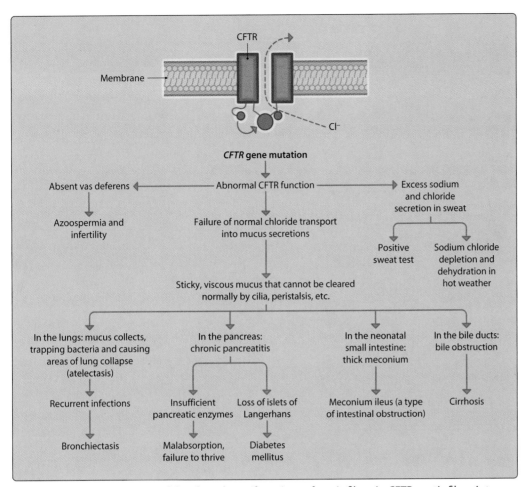

Fig. 3.50.1 Pathophysiology of the clinical manifestations of cystic fibrosis. CFTR, cystic fibrosis transmembrane conductance regulator.

CFTR controls the transport of chloride ions across cell membranes by providing a channel through which they can move; it also appears to regulate other transmembrane transporters. Normally, mucus-secreting cells transport chloride out of the cytoplasm into the secreted mucus; sodium ions and water follow passively, keeping the mucus moist. The molecular basis of the abnormality in cystic fibrosis is not fully understood, but impaired transport of chloride out of the cytoplasm creates sticky, viscous mucus secretions in the pancreas, lungs and other organs (Fig. 3.50.1). In addition, the vasa deferentia are commonly absent in males. The sweat of patients with cystic fibrosis has abnormally *high* concentrations of sodium and chloride ions, and the finding of excessively salty sweat is the basis of a diagnostic test for cystic fibrosis.

Alcoholism. The commonest cause of chronic pancreatitis is chronic alcoholism. In alcoholics, chronic pancreatitis is frequently a relapsing condition in which episodes of acute pancreatitis occur intermittently, each one causing further pancreatic damage.

Autoimmune chronic pancreatitis. This unusual condition is characterized by damage to ducts by a chronic inflammatory infiltrate composed mainly of lymphocytes. Patients may also have other autoimmune diseases.

Chronic obstruction. Pseudocysts, neoplasms and anatomical abnormalities may cause chronic pancreatitis. However, chronic pancreatitis caused by gallstones is relatively uncommon—gallstones tend to be associated with acute pancreatitis.

Cystic fibrosis (mucoviscidosis). This condition is an autosomal recessive defect in the cystic fibrosis transmembrane conductance regulator (CFTR) encoded by the gene *CFTR*.

Hereditary chronic pancreatitis. Abnormalities in a number of different genes have been identified as causes of hereditary chronic pancreatitis. Interestingly, some patients have abnormalities of *CFTR* although they do not have features typical of cystic fibrosis.

Pathology

The pancreas is firm because of fibrosis, and the ducts are often dilated and contain protein plugs. Atrophy of the exocrine tissue occurs and results in malabsorption through loss of pancreatic enzyme production. Often, the endocrine tissue of the islets of Langerhans is preserved until late in the disease, but eventually the islets, too, may be destroyed; the result is diabetes mellitus. Foci of calcification are common and there may be pseudocyst formation. Abdominal pain is the most common presenting feature, sometimes in the context of an acute exacerbation of the inflammation.

51. Diabetes mellitus: pathophysiology

Questions
- What are the functions of insulin?
- What are the differences between types 1 and 2 diabetes mellitus?

Diabetes mellitus is a chronic disorder caused by inadequate insulin action; this can arise either from impaired insulin production or from resistance of target organs to insulin action. There are consequent abnormalities of carbohydrate, fat and protein metabolism. Its hallmark is hyperglycaemia (increased blood glucose concentration). This chapter covers the pathophysiology; the complications of diabetes are described in Ch. 52.

Insulin

Insulin is secreted by the beta cells of the islets of Langerhans in response to a rise in blood glucose. When insulin binds to the insulin receptor on the surface of a cell it initiates a number of anabolic processes:

- transmembrane transport of glucose into muscle, fat and other tissues
- glycogen synthesis from glucose in muscle and liver
- conversion of glucose into fat
- transmembrane transport of amino acids into muscle and other tissues
- protein synthesis in muscle and other tissues.

It also inhibits the use of fats and proteins for energy. The net result is that the concentration of glucose in the blood tends to fall (hypoglycaemic effect). Insulin is the only hormone in the body that has this effect, whereas there are several hormones that tend to have a hyperglycaemic effect, and the hyperglycaemic actions of these hormones cannot be adequately opposed if insulin action is deficient (Fig. 3.51.1).

Consequently, the major effects of insulin deficiency are catabolic: that is, there is breakdown of energy stores in the tissues. Lipolysis converts fats into free fatty acids and glycerol; proteins are broken down into amino acids, which are then used for glucose production (gluconeogenesis), and glycogen is cleaved into glucose molecules. Thus, the excess circulating glucose in diabetics is derived from ingested glucose that cannot be taken up by the cells and also from the breakdown of alternative energy stores (fat, glycogen and protein; Fig. 3.51.1).

Pathogenesis

Diabetes mellitus is not a single disease but a condition found in a number of heterogeneous disorders. Current classifications divide diabetes mellitus into type 1, type 2, and other specific types.

Type 1 diabetes

Type 1 diabetes is characterized by inadequate insulin secretion by the islets of Langerhans. Patients usually need insulin injections to control their blood sugar levels, and it is diagnosed before age 35 years in the great majority.

Most cases result from autoimmune destruction of beta cells, although in a few instances there is no demonstrable autoimmunity and the pathogenesis is obscure. The autoimmune injury is thought to be mediated principally by T-cells, and in many cases a lymphocytic inflammation of the islets (so-called **insulitis**) can be observed. There is some evidence that viral infection (e.g. mumps or coxsackievirus) can initiate or promote the autoimmune reaction. Other organ-specific autoimmune diseases such as Hashimoto thyroiditis, Graves' disease, coeliac disease, Addison's disease and pernicious anaemia occur in approximately 10–20% of type 1 diabetics.

Type 2 diabetes

Type 2 is the most common type of diabetes, accounting for approximately 90% of those with diabetes. It classically presents in middle age, but increasingly it is appearing in younger individuals, obese children in particular.

The central defect is failure of target cells to respond adequately to stimulation by insulin (insulin resistance). The mechanism is unclear, but obesity is an important risk factor, and there is growing evidence that insulin resistance can be promoted by various hormones secreted by adipose tissue, such as resistin and leptin.

In early type 2 diabetes, insulin levels are commonly elevated to counteract the insulin resistance of target organs. Later in the course of the disease, this compensatory increase in insulin secretion fails,

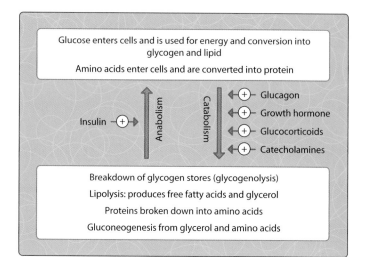

Fig. 3.51.1 Anabolic and catabolic hormones.

and an absolute deficiency of insulin supervenes. It seems that the beta cells become unresponsive to the signal provided by elevated glucose. An intriguing observation is that most type 2 diabetics have amyloid deposition in the islets, and it is possible that this amyloid could contribute to failure of beta cell function.

In some cases, type 2 diabetes is associated with **metabolic syndrome X**, also called **insulin resistance syndrome**. Metabolic syndrome X is not a type of diabetes, but many individuals with it also have type 2 diabetes because of the insulin resistance and consequent glucose intolerance. Metabolic syndrome X is a complex constellation of metabolic abnormalities, including:

- central obesity, i.e. obesity of the abdomen and/or viscera
- hypertension
- insulin resistance with glucose intolerance and compensatory hyperinsulinaemia
- increased sympathetic nervous activity
- dyslipidaemia (increased circulating triglyceride and low density lipoproteins, and reduced circulating high density lipoproteins)
- abnormalities of clotting and fibrinolysis associated with abnormal circulating levels of clotting and fibrinolytic factors and endothelial cell dysfunction.

Metabolic syndrome X is a common condition in industrialized countries and affects approximately a quarter of adults in the USA. Its importance is that it is associated with a particularly high risk of atherosclerosis.

Other types of diabetes mellitus

Pancreatic diseases that damage the islets of Langerhans can cause diabetes, for example pancreatitis, haemochromatosis, cystic fibrosis and surgical removal of the pancreas.

Hyperglycaemia can occur if there is an excess of diabetogenic hormones. For example, steroid therapy and Cushing's syndrome are associated with excess glucocorticoids; there is excess growth hormone in acromegaly; and excess glucagon and catecholamines in glucagonoma and phaeochromocytoma, respectively.

In pregnancy, there is a tendency to insulin resistance and thus diabetes may be 'unmasked' in pregnant women and then may persist after delivery. The term **gestational diabetes** is used

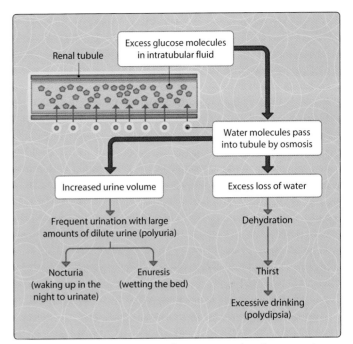

Fig. 3.51.2 The pathogenesis of symptoms related to osmotic diuresis in diabetes mellitus.

when the condition occurs during pregnancy and then disappears after childbirth.

Certain rare genetic defects of insulin production or the insulin receptor cause diabetes. In addition, hyperglycaemia is common in Down's syndrome.

Consequences of inadequate insulin action

Diabetes mellitus is defined by the presence of hyperglycaemia. When the plasma concentration of glucose exceeds approximately 11 mmol/l, glucose appears in the urine (**glycosuria**). Indeed, the term diabetes mellitus comes from the Greek words for 'running through' and 'sweet' on account of the sugar in the urine. The excess glucose in the renal tubules causes an osmotic diuresis, which is responsible for many of the symptoms of diabetes mellitus (Fig. 3.51.2).

Because fats and proteins are broken down for energy, the body enters a catabolic state. Weight loss is the result, even though appetite is stimulated and the patient eats more (**polyphagia**).

52. Diabetes mellitus: complications

Questions
- What are the acute complications of diabetes mellitus?
- What are the long-term complications?
- What infectious complications of diabetes mellitus can occur?

For ease of discussion, complications are divided into three groups: acute, chronic and infectious.

Acute complications

Diabetic ketoacidosis. Lipolysis is a characteristic of insulin lack (Ch. 51). Released free fatty acids are converted in the liver to ketone bodies (e.g. acetoacetate, acetone and 3-hydroxybutyrate). These substances are acidic and release hydrogen ions, causing metabolic acidosis. The combination of excess ketone bodies (ketosis) and acidosis is called ketoacidosis, and is usually seen in type 1 diabetes.

Hyperosmolar non-ketotic syndrome. This condition typically occurs in older patients with type 2 diabetes. It is characterized by hyperglycaemia and dehydration. A typical scenario is a patient who does not drink enough water to compensate for the urinary losses through osmotic diuresis; the consequence is a rise in serum osmolality. Ketoacidosis is minimal or absent.

Lactic acidosis. Rarely, diabetics present with lactic acidosis. The prognosis is poor.

Hypoglycaemia. This is a complication seen in treated diabetics who take insulin (or occasionally other hypoglycaemic agents) in excess of requirements. The resultant fall in blood glucose can cause mental symptoms, hunger, palpitations, sweating, abnormalities of behaviour and convulsions. In severe hypoglycaemia, patients may present with coma, but this must not be confused with the coma caused by ketoacidosis in untreated diabetes.

Chronic complications

Diabetes is one of the most important causes of morbidity and mortality in the industrialized world, largely through its effects on blood vessels (atheroma and microangiopathy). Coronary artery disease, cerebrovascular events, peripheral vascular disease and renal failure are common in diabetics; approximately 80% of adult diabetics die from cardiovascular disease. Furthermore, long-standing diabetes mellitus, especially type 1, is often complicated by serious retinal disease. Most of these complications appear to be directly related to hyperglycaemia, and good control of blood glucose levels delays their development. The mechanisms linking hyperglycaemia to these complications are only partially understood, but the following appear to be important.

Glycosylation of proteins. Glucose can bind to proteins by chemical reactions that do not depend on enzymes (non-enzymatic glycosylation), and this process may be important in the pathogenesis of diabetic complications (Fig. 3.52.1). The amount of non-enzymatically glycosylated protein in the body is directly proportional to the level of blood glucose. This phenomenon is exploited in the glycosylated haemoglobin (HbA1c) test, in which the level of circulating HbA1c is used as a measure of the average blood glucose over the previous few weeks, and thus as an indication of the control of blood glucose achieved by a diabetic patient.

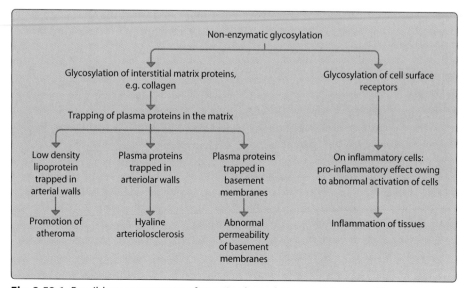

Fig. 3.52.1 Possible consequences of protein glycosylation in diabetes mellitus.

Polyol pathway disruption. In diabetics, intracellular hyperglycaemia occurs in those cells that do not require insulin for glucose transport (e.g. nerves, lens, kidney). The excess glucose is metabolized to sorbitol (a polyol), which is then converted to fructose. The sorbitol and fructose increase intracellular osmolality, causing osmotic influx of water and cellular swelling. Sorbitol also impairs the function of ion pumps. These processes are believed to be important in the development of, for example, diabetic retinopathy, diabetic neuropathy and cataracts.

Hypertension. Many diabetics (over half of them in some studies) have hypertension, which acts synergistically with other mechanisms to promote atheroma.

Vascular disease

Vascular complications of diabetes can be divided into disease of large vessels (i.e. **atherosclerosis**) and disease of small vessels (i.e. **diabetic microangiopathy**). The atherosclerosis in diabetics is morphologically indistinguishable from that which occurs in non-diabetics (Ch. 34) but the process is accelerated and the lesions occur at an earlier age. Diabetic microangiopathy is characterized morphologically by hyaline arteriolosclerosis and diffuse thickening of basement membranes.

Kidney disease (diabetic nephropathy)

The vascular complications of diabetes have important effects in the kidneys (Fig. 3.52.2). Large-vessel disease causes renal artery atherosclerosis, which can reduce the flow of blood through the kidney. Microangiopathy causes hyaline arteriolosclerosis of the afferent and efferent arterioles and thickening and abnormal permeability of glomerular basement membranes. This change in permeability allows the glomeruli to leak plasma proteins into the filtrate and these proteins are lost in the urine (proteinuria).

Ocular complications

Diabetes is a common cause of visual impairment or blindness. The principal lesions responsible are:

- **retinopathy**: retinal changes may be non-proliferative or proliferative; non-proliferative retinopathy includes haemorrhages, exudates, microaneurysms, thickening of retinal capillaries and oedema; proliferative retinopathy arises from neovascularization (new blood vessel formation) and fibrosis
- **cataract**: damage to the crystalline lens
- **glaucoma**: in advanced disease, a network of new vessels may form a ring at the margin of the pupil and in the anterior chamber, causing closed-angle glaucoma.

Diabetic neuropathy

Peripheral neuropathy may involve the sensory, motor and autonomic nerves. The pathogenesis is not well understood, but microangiopathy, protein glycosylation and intracellular hyperglycaemia could all be involved.

Infectious complications

Diabetics are more prone to certain infections than normal individuals and in approximately 5% infection is the cause of death. The pathogenesis of the increased susceptibility is multifactorial and can include a number of different processes. For example, neutrophil function is impaired in diabetics, and poor blood supply in accompanying vascular disease predisposes to infection and inhibits healing. In body fluids (especially the urine), the abnormal presence of glucose can promote the growth of bacteria.

Common infectious complications of diabetes include skin infections (e.g. boils and foot ulcers), pneumonia, urinary tract infection, vaginal candidiasis and tuberculosis. Additionally, diabetics are predisposed to **mucormycosis**, an unusual fungal infection by members of the zygomycetes, principally *Mucor*, that occurs in diabetics and the immunosuppressed. It involves the paranasal sinuses and the lungs and can spread to the brain to produce a serious meningoencephalitis.

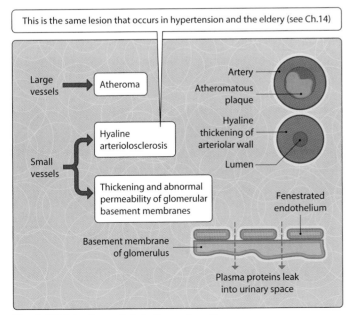

Fig. 3.52.2 Lesions of diabetic angiopathy.

53. Fatty change and cirrhosis

Questions
- What are the main causes of fatty change within the liver?
- What is cirrhosis and what are its major causes?
- What are the complications of cirrhosis?

Fatty change

Fatty change (**steatosis**) is the most common response of the liver to injury. Morphologically, it is characterized by the accumulation of globules of lipid within the cytoplasm of hepatocytes. In most cases, the globules enlarge and coalesce until the nucleus and cytoplasm of the cell are displaced to the periphery; this is known as **macrovesicular steatosis** (Fig. 3.53.1). In **microvesicular steatosis**, the globules all remain small. There are many causes of fatty change, including ethanol, drugs, toxins, diabetes mellitus, obesity, hypertriglyceridaemia, protein malnutrition, total parenteral nutrition and severe systemic illnesses.

Fatty change accompanied by inflammatory changes is **steatohepatitis** (Fig. 3.53.2), which is characterized by infiltration of the parenchyma by neutrophils, swelling of hepatocytes (ballooning degeneration), and Mallory bodies, which are tangles of intermediate filaments and ubiquitin, seen on H&E stained sections as bright pink hyaline inclusions. Collagen production by stellate cells causes fibrosis (Fig. 3.53.3), which can progress to cirrhosis.

The most common cause of fatty change and steatohepatitis in industrialized countries is chronic alcoholism; the diseases are called alcoholic fatty change and alcoholic steatohepatitis, respectively, whereas those caused by conditions other than ethanol toxicity are called non-alcoholic fatty change and non-alcoholic steatohepatitis (NASH), respectively. The commonest cause of NASH is metabolic syndrome (Ch. 51). Fatty change is completely reversible, provided the aetiology is eliminated. Steatohepatitis is also reversible, provided the fibrosis is not too far advanced.

Pathogenesis

The pathways involved in fatty change are complex and only partially understood, but in principle triglycerides accumulate in the liver because of either increased synthesis from free fatty acids within hepatocytes or decreased export as very low density lipoproteins. In fatty liver induced by certain toxins, decreased oxidation of free fatty acids may contribute to their accumulation. Impaired synthesis of apolipoproteins (lipid-binding proteins in lipoproteins) is seen in many types of fatty liver, including that caused by malnutrition.

Ethanol could damage the liver in a number of ways. It is oxidized in the liver to acetaldehyde, which is potentially toxic, and its metabolism also produces reduced nicotinamide adenine dinucleotide (NADH), which promotes a reduced intracellular condition (increased redox state) that interferes with many aspects of intermediary metabolism. Furthermore, free radicals are produced during ethanol metabolism, and ethanol itself appears to impair microtubular function. Other factors may act synergistically with ethanol to promote liver damage. For example, people who drink large amounts of alcohol often neglect other aspects of their diet, because the alcohol itself is a major source of calories, and may lack certain nutritional factors (such as vitamin B_{12}), thus compounding the effects of alcohol.

Cirrhosis

Cirrhosis is defined as nodules of regenerating hepatocytes surrounded by fibrous septa and affecting the liver diffusely. It is the final common pathway for many different types of liver injury. Worldwide, the principal causes are alcoholic liver

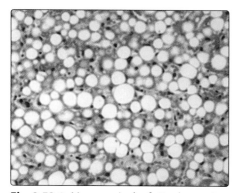

Fig. 3.53.1 Macrovesicular fatty change in a patient with chronic alcoholism.

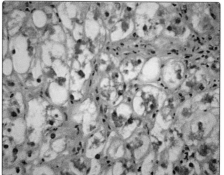

Fig. 3.53.2 Alcoholic steatohepatitis. The hepatocytes show ballooning degeneration and many contain Mallory bodies.

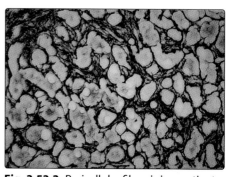

Fig. 3.53.3 Pericellular fibrosis in a patient with alchoholic liver disease. This reticulin stain demonstrates the increased amounts of collagen in the perisinusoidal spaces.

disease and chronic viral hepatitis. Other common causes include non-alcoholic steatohepatitis, biliary tract diseases and haemochromatosis. The term cryptogenic cirrhosis is used for those patients in whom no specific cause is identified.

Pathophysiology

The damage to the liver causes cytokine production by Kupffer cells and other inflammatory cells. These cytokines induce inflammation and also activate stellate cells (or Ito cells), which reside in the perisinusoidal space of Disse. The normal function of stellate cells is to store vitamin A. However, when activated, they take on the characteristics of myofibroblasts and synthesize matrix material, as a result of which collagen and other matrix substances are deposited in the space of Disse (Fig. 3.53.3). **Perisinusoidal fibrosis**, exacerbated by contraction of the myofibroblast-like stellate cells, increases resistance to blood flow and causes portal hypertension. Thrombosis of veins also increases resistance to intrahepatic blood flow. Meanwhile, loss of hepatocytes by apoptosis and necrosis results in mitotic activity of hepatocytes (hepatocellular regeneration).

The normal sinusoidal endothelium is fenestrated, but as cirrhosis develops the endothelium loses its fenestrations in a process called **capillarization of sinusoids**. The capillarization and perisinusoidal fibrosis inhibit the exchange of solutes between the hepatocytes and the blood, thus impairing the secretion of proteins synthesized by the liver (e.g. albumin, clotting factors).

As the process continues, the fibrosis tends to concentrate in areas of greatest cell damage and forms band-like scars (septa) that separate nodules of hepatocytes. At this stage, the liver has become cirrhotic. Important changes in the microanatomy of the liver vasculature occur as the fibrous scars grow. Abnormal shunts develop between the portal veins and the hepatic arteries and hepatic veins. These shunts allow blood to bypass the hepatocytes, compromising the ability of the liver to detoxify the blood. The abnormal circulation and capillarization of sinusoids in cirrhotic livers deprive hepatocytes of nutrients and oxygen, causing further hepatocyte injury. The pathogenetic mechanisms leading to cirrhosis are summarized in Fig. 3.53.4.

Clinical effects

Many patients with cirrhosis are asymptomatic or have only mild, non-specific constitutional symptoms such as anorexia. If significant clinical features occur, they are likely to be caused by liver failure, portal hypertension and/or the development of hepatocellular carcinoma.

Liver failure results when the various metabolic functions of the liver are sufficiently impaired; clinical features include jaundice, reduced production of albumin and clotting factors, and itching owing to accumulation of bile salts in the skin. Portal hypertension causes accumulation of fluid in the abdomen (**ascites**) because of increased hydrostatic pressure in the portal veins; ascites may be exacerbated by hypoalbuminaemia in liver failure. Portal hypertension also causes increased flow where the portal and systemic circulations anastomose (i.e. lower oesophagus, rectum and anterior abdominal wall; the last via the umbilical vein), and the veins in these places become tortuous and dilated. The dilated oesophageal veins (**oesophageal varices**) are prone to rupture. Chronic congestion of the spleen in portal hypertension causes **splenomegaly**.

Hepatocellular carcinoma can arise in any form of cirrhosis. However, some aetiologies (e.g. haemochromatosis) seem more likely to be complicated by hepatocellular carcinoma.

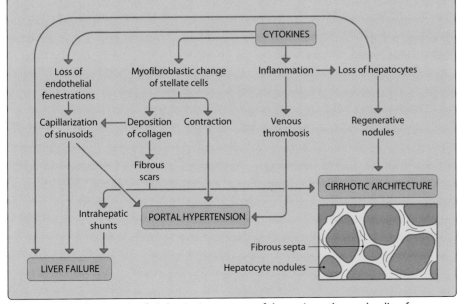

Fig. 3.53.4 Pathogenesis of cirrhosis. A summary of the main pathways leading from cytokine production in the damaged liver to the architectural changes of cirrhosis, liver failure and portal hypertension.

54. Urinary tract infection

Questions
- What are the main risk factors for the development of urinary tract infection?
- What is the difference between acute and chronic pyelonephritis?

Infection of the urinary tract is a common disease. If it involves the kidneys, it can cause renal failure. Normally, the bladder and upper urinary tract are sterile, although commensal organisms are found in the distal urethra. Host defence mechanisms that keep the bladder and upper urinary tract free of infection include regular evacuation of the bladder, which helps to eliminate any organisms that gain access to the bladder lumen; tight junctions between cells of the transitional epithelium, which act as a mechanical barrier; and resident inflammatory cells in the mucosa, including plasma cells that secrete IgA.

Aetiology and pathogenesis

By far the most common route of infection is via the urethra. These ascending infections are caused by organisms derived from the patient's own faecal commensals that gain access to the urethra. *Escherichia coli* is the most frequent, but any faecal organism can be responsible. Sometimes, sexually transmitted organisms such as *Neisseria gonorrhoeae* cause ascending infections.

Any of the factors that predispose to infection in general increase the risk of urinary tract infection (Ch. 16). There are also factors specific to the urinary tract, which will predispose to ascending infection (Fig. 3.54.1).

Stasis of urine. If there is incomplete emptying of the bladder at each micturition, there will be a failure to clear the bladder of any contaminating organisms. This occurs in bladder outflow obstruction, as seen in urethral stricture, bladder tumours at the internal urethral orifice and nodular hyperplasia of the prostate, or when the nerve supply to the bladder is interrupted thus preventing normal contraction of the detrusor muscle.

Foreign body. The most common foreign body in clinical practice is a urinary catheter. Like any foreign body, a catheter can act as a focus for infection by providing a site where bacteria can multiply in a place protected from host defence mechanisms. Furthermore, catheterization can introduce microorganisms from the anterior urethra into the bladder. Another structure that can act as a foreign body is a urinary stone. Whether in the bladder or upper urinary tract, stones can act as a nidus of infection.

Alkaline urine. In general, an acidic environment inhibits the growth of pathogenic bacteria. Therefore, bacteria are able to multiply in urine more readily if it is alkaline.

Female sex. Urinary tract infections are much more common in females. This phenomenon can be ascribed to the relatively short female urethra, allowing easier migration from the exterior of the body into the bladder.

Adherence by microorganisms. Bacteria that can cause urinary tract infections generally have the ability to adhere to the transitional epithelium of the urinary tract, enabled by adhesion molecules (adhesins) on the fimbriae of the bacteria.

Lower urinary tract infection

Infections of the urethra and bladder cause **urethritis** and **cystitis**, respectively. The pathological changes are those typical of inflammation, with hyperaemia, oedema and accumulation of inflammatory cells. If the oedema is very pronounced, the mucosa is thrown into folds that bulge into the bladder lumen, forming polyps; the condition is called **polypoid cystitis**. (A polyp is any structure that stands up from a mucosal surface. It should not be confused with the term papilloma, which specifically refers to a polyp with a fibrovascular core covered by epithelium.) Sometimes, small cysts form in the inflamed bladder mucosa, a condition that pathologists call **cystitis cystica**. If the inflammation is chronic, the transitional epithelium of the bladder can show metaplastic change and transform either into mucus-secreting glandular epithelium (called **cystitis glandularis**) or into keratinizing squamous epithelium. The latter is more likely when there is chronic irritation of the mucosa, for example in schistosomiasis.

Occasionally, the bladder exhibits an unusual inflammatory reaction called **malacoplakia.** This condition can occur at many different sites in the body, but the renal tract is one of the places where it is seen more often. Malacoplakia is a granulomatous inflammation in which large macrophages with granular cytoplasm containing round calcified bodies are prominent. Macroscopically, it produces a soft, pale yellow lesion. Xanthogranulomatous inflammation is a similar condition, but the macrophages are foamier and the calcified bodies are absent.

Pyelonephritis

Infection of the kidney and its collecting system (i.e. upper urinary tract infection) is termed pyelonephritis. It can be acute or chronic. There are two main routes of infection (Fig. 3.54.1).

The most common pathway is **ascending infection** from the lower urinary tract. In order for bacteria to gain access to the

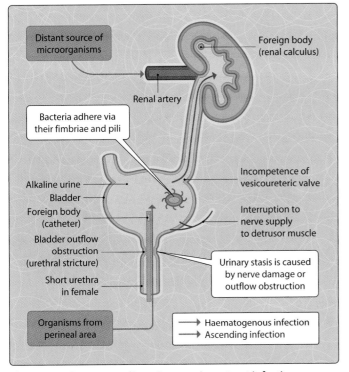

Fig. 3.54.1 Factors predisposing to urinary tract infection.

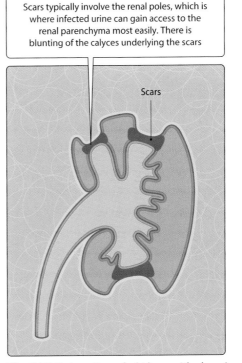

Fig. 3.54.3 A section of a kidney with chronic pyelonephritis.

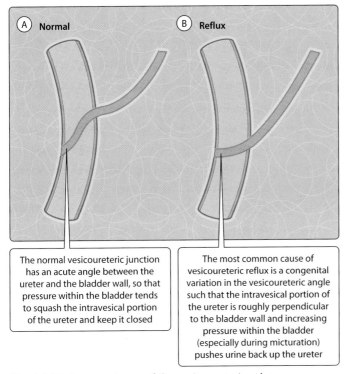

Fig. 3.54.2 Incompetence of the vesicoureteric valve.

ureter from the bladder, there must be incompetence of the vesicoureteric valve, allowing reflux of urine into the ureter (Fig. 3.54.2). In the absence of reflux, the infection usually remains confined to the bladder. However, vesicoureteric reflux is common, and any patient with infective cystitis should be considered potentially at risk of developing pyelonephritis.

Occasionally, pyelonephritis is caused by **haematogenous spread** of bacteria from elsewhere in the body. For example, the kidneys can be seeded with bacteria during septicaemia or infective endocarditis, and tuberculous pyelonephritis can result from spread of tubercle bacilli from a distant site, usually the lungs. Although direct spread from adjacent tissues can theoretically occur, and thus be a third possible route of infection, in practice this is a rare occurrence.

Acute pyelonephritis causes suppurative inflammation of the kidney. If the pelvicalyceal system fills with pus, the term **pyonephrosis** is used. A potentially serious complication that occurs in severe cases is papillary necrosis. In this condition, the distal portions of the renal pyramids show coagulative necrosis. Acute renal failure may follow. If the necrotic papillae break off completely, they can obstruct the ureter. Although most patients recover from acute pyelonephritis, there is a risk that the disease can progress to chronic pyelonephritis.

Chronic pyelonephritis implies chronic inflammation of the kidney and is associated with the formation of scars in the renal parenchyma (Fig. 3.54.3). Histologically, the scars show atrophy and fibrosis of the renal tissue and variable numbers of chronic inflammatory cells. In some patients, the presentation is with secondary hypertension caused by the renal damage whereas in others, chronic renal failure follows loss of functioning renal tissue.

55. Glomerulonephritis

Questions
- What is glomerulonephritis?
- What are the pathological mechanisms involved in its development?
- What are the clinical sequelae of glomerulonephritis?

Glomerular injury is an important cause of renal failure. The term glomerulonephritis is used rather loosely for any disease process affecting the glomeruli, although processes in which there is no infiltrate of inflammatory cells are sometimes called glomerulopathies. Sometimes, the glomerular injury can be the primary disease process, but glomerulonephritis can also occur as a complication of other conditions, in which case the term secondary glomerulonephritis can be used. Secondary glomerulonephritis is common and is seen in a wide variety of different diseases, including diabetes mellitus, hypertension and systemic lupus erythematosus.

Renal biopsy is commonly used in the investigation of glomerulonephritis because the pattern of glomerular injury can be a clue to the aetiology and/or prognosis.

Mechanisms of glomerular injury

The pathogenesis of glomerulonephritis can be immunological or non-immunological.

Immunological mechanisms

The primary glomerulonephritides and many of the secondary glomerulonephritides are caused by the presence of immunoglobulin within the glomerulus and are, therefore, said to be immune mediated (Fig. 3.55.1). The processes involved are only partially understood. It is helpful to think of them in two main groups: immune complex deposition and nephrotoxic antibody.

Immune complex deposition
Immune complexes are formed when immunoglobulin and antigen clump together to form insoluble particles. When immunofluorescence is used to detect the presence of these immune complexes in renal biopsies, a granular appearance is seen. Most immunologically mediated glomerulonephritides are of this type.

Within the circulation, these particles can become trapped in capillaries (Fig. 3.55.1A). When deposited in this way, the immune complexes activate inflammatory cells and initiate the complement cascade, causing inflammation. The glomerulus is a common site for immune complex entrapment, so glomerulonephritis is a common phenomenon when circulating immune complexes are present. The pattern of injury depends on the site of the immune complex deposition and the modifying effects of T-cells.

A similar process occurs when immune complexes form in situ within the glomerulus, For example, antigenic material can collect in the glomerulus (planted antigen) and then the binding of antibody produces immune complexes (Fig. 3.55.1B).

Post-infective glomerulonephritis occurs when immunoglobulin forms complexes with an antigen derived from a microorganism. For example, in post-streptococcal glomerulonephritis, immune complexes are deposited in the glomeruli approximately 7–14 days after infection with certain strains of β-haemolytic streptococci. The consequent glomerulonephritis typically causes the nephritic syndrome (see below). Whether the antigens are planted in the glomerulus or are derived from circulating immune complexes (or both) is not known.

Nephrotoxic antibody
An autoimmune reaction directed against a native component of the glomerular basement membrane results in diffuse binding of IgG (Fig. 3.55.1C). On immunofluorescence, this process is characterized by a linear appearance, rather than the granular deposition seen with immune complexes. The condition is known as **antiglomerular basement membrane disease**. It accounts for less than 5% of all primary glomerulonephritis. It occurs in Goodpasture syndrome, in which the glomerulonephritis is associated with pulmonary haemorrhage because the antigen is also found in the basement membranes of alveoli. There is binding of IgG to the alveoli, identical to the process occurring in the glomeruli, with consequent activation of inflammatory cells and initiation of the complement cascade.

Non-immunological mechanisms

Some secondary glomerular lesions are not primarily immunological, for example in hypertension, amyloidosis and diabetes mellitus. Diabetic glomerulosclerosis is described in Ch. 52.

Hypertension causes narrowing of arteries through medial and intimal thickening, and narrowing of arterioles through hyaline arteriolosclerosis; the overall result is reduced blood flow to the glomeruli and it is the resulting glomerular ischaemia that causes the damage. A kidney affected by hypertension in this way shows atrophy of the renal parenchyma and fibrosis of glomeruli (**glomerulosclerosis**).

Involvement of the kidney is common in systemic amyloidosis. The amyloid is deposited not only in the walls of glomeruli and other blood vessels but also the interstitium.

Clinical manifestations of glomerular injury

Glomerular disease produces five main syndromes:

Nephrotic syndrome. The hallmark of the nephrotic syndrome is marked proteinuria (>3.5 g per day). The liver is unable to replace all the albumin lost in the urine, so there is hypoalbuminaemia. The hypoalbuminaemia causes a fall in plasma oncotic pressure, which causes oedema. There is also hyperlipidaemia.

Nephritic syndrome. This is characterized by haematuria, hypertension and acute renal failure with reduced urine output. In contrast to the nephrotic syndrome, proteinuria is usually mild.

Recurrent painless haematuria. Haematuria may be macroscopic (visible to the patient) or microscopic (detected only on testing the urine).

Asymptomatic proteinuria. This is loss of protein found on testing the urine in a patient who has no symptoms.

Chronic renal failure. If the glomerular damage is severe and irreversible, chronic renal failure occurs. It can be associated with failure of erythropoietin production, which causes anaemia. Abnormalities of bone metabolism may occur, causing skeletal abnormalities called renal osteodystrophy (Ch. 59). The pathophysiology of renal osteodystrophy is complex, but central to its causation is failure of the kidney to process vitamin D (which results in hypocalcaemia) and failure of the kidney to excrete excess phosphate (which produces hyperphosphataemia).

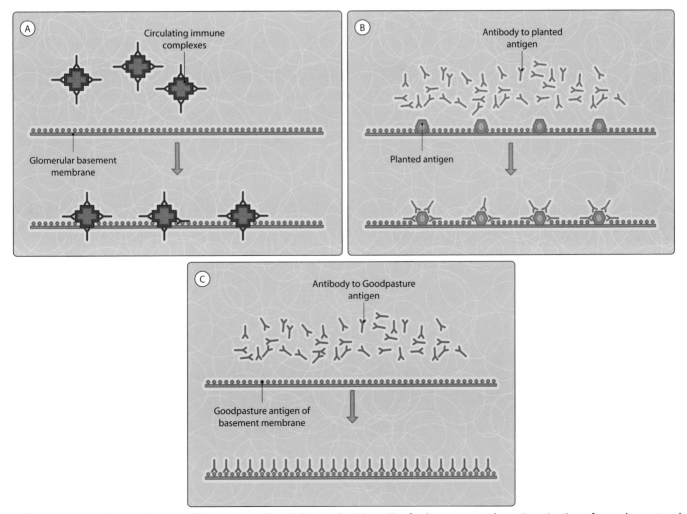

Fig. 3.55.1 The three main types of immune-mediated glomerular injury. The final common pathway is activation of complement and inflammatory cells. (A) Circulating immune complexes are trapped in the glomeruli. (B) Antibodies to a 'planted' antigen cause in-situ immune complex formation. (C) Nephrotoxic antibody: antiglomerular basement membrane immunoglobulin binds to the basement membrane in a linear fashion.

56. Raised intracranial pressure

Questions
- What are the major causes of raised intracranial pressure?
- What are the clinical sequelae?
- What are the pathological intracranial consequences of a head injury?

The brain and spinal cord are enclosed by a rigid compartment, namely the skull and vertebral bodies. Although these bony structures serve to protect the delicate tissues of the central nervous system (CNS), any increase in the volume of the tissues within them is accompanied by an increase in pressure.

Causes of increased intracranial pressure

The pressure of the cerebrospinal fluid (CSF) is normally <15 mmHg (lower in children). Table 3.56.1 lists causes of raised intracranial pressure. Many different injuries to the CNS are associated with oedema of the parenchyma. Injury to brain cells causes defects in ion transport, allowing fluid to enter cells, and disruption of the integrity of the blood–brain barrier allows fluid to escape from the blood into the interstitial space. Oedematous brain is soft and the sulci are narrowed.

Effects of raised intracranial pressure

There are two important complications of raised intracranial pressure: **herniation** and **reduced cerebral blood flow.**

Pressure gradients within the skull can cause brain tissue to herniate across the dural reflections or into the foramen magnum (Fig. 3.56.1). In **subfalcine herniation**, the cingulate gyrus is pushed under the falx cerebri. As a consequence, branches of the anterior cerebral artery may be compressed, causing ischaemic injury that often involves the sensory and motor cortex supplying the lower limbs. **Transtentorial (uncinate) herniation** usually involves the medial aspect of the temporal lobe (uncus), which is pushed inferiorly around the unyielding tentorium cerebelli. The third cranial nerve is compressed, causing signs of a third cranial nerve palsy. Pressure on the posterior cerebral artery can cause ischaemic injury to the visual cortex. **Tonsillar herniation** compresses the brainstem and the vital centres therein and is a life-threatening emergency. A common complication of tonsillar herniation is haemorrhagic lesions of the brainstem; they are believed to be haemorrhagic infarcts as a result of compression of branches of the basilar artery.

When intracranial pressure exceeds approximately 30 mmHg, the normal systemic arterial pressure is unable to force sufficient blood into the cranial cavity. Systemic blood pressure rises while heart rate and respiratory rate fall, tending to preserve cerebral perfusion (the Cushing reflex). However, if intracerebral pressure rises sufficiently, these compensatory mechanisms will be unable to maintain cerebral arterial perfusion, the cerebral blood flow becomes inadequate, and diffuse neuronal injury follows.

Table 3.56.1 CAUSES OF RAISED INTRACRANIAL PRESSURE

	Type	Examples
Local mass (space-occupying lesion)	Non-neoplastic Neoplastic	Haemorrhage; abscess Primary brain tumour; metastasis
Focal oedema	Surrounding a lesion Surrounding tissue damaged by penetrating trauma	Tumour; infarct; abscess Bullet or shrapnel wounds
Diffuse oedema	Traumatic diffuse neuronal injury Widespread inflammation Hypoxia Toxic effects	Shaken brain syndrome Meningitis; encephalitis; subarachnoid haemorrhage Shock Lead poisoning; some antibiotics
Intracranial congestion	Obstruction to venous outflow	Dural sinus thrombosis
Hydrocephalus (increase in CSF)	Obstruction to CSF flow or prevention of resorption of CSF at arachnoid granulations Increased production of CSF (rare)	Intraventricular haemorrhage; subarachnoid haemorrhage; meningitis Tumour of choroid plexus
Idiopathic		Benign intracranial hypertension

CSF, cerebrospinal fluid.

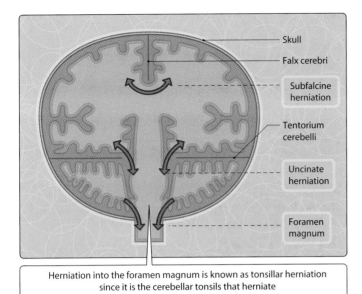

Herniation into the foramen magnum is known as tonsillar herniation since it is the cerebellar tonsils that herniate

Fig. 3.56.1 Types of cerebral herniation shown in a coronal section to demonstrate herniation beneath the falx cerebri, across the tentorium cerebelli and into the foramen magnum. The last is called tonsillar herniation since it is the cerebellar tonsils that herniate.

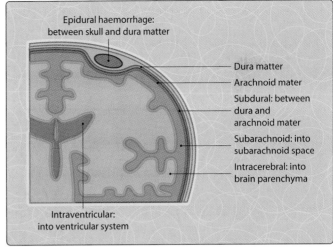

Fig. 3.56.2 Sites of intracranial haemorrhage. This coronal section shows a small epidural (extradural) haemorrhage. The other possible compartments into which haemorrhage can occur are also shown.

Traumatic brain injury

Head trauma can injure the brain in different ways.

Intracranial haemorrhage. Such a haemorrhage will act as a space-occupying lesion (Fig. 3.56.2). Epidural (extradural) haematoma usually results from a skull fracture that tears a meningeal artery or one of its branches. The commonest scenario is a fracture of the squamous temporal bone associated with rupture of the middle meningeal artery. Subdural haematomas are usually caused by rupture of the bridging veins that connect intracerebral veins to the dural sinuses. They are often associated with acceleration/deceleration injuries, which cause the brain to move relative to the skull. Atrophic brains are more mobile within the cranial cavity and are thus more prone to subdural haematoma; in some cases the trauma causing the haemorrhage may be so minor it is not noticed.

Contusions. Bruises caused by blunt trauma most commonly occur in the superficial brain parenchyma when the brain and the skull collide. A common occurrence in this respect is the presence of coup and contrecoup injuries. The coup injury is contusion in the brain immediately under the blow that caused it. However, movement of the brain within the skull may bring the opposite pole of the brain into contact with bone, causing a contrecoup (opposite the blow) injury. For example, consider the case of someone falling backwards so their occiput strikes a hard floor. Contusions of the occipital lobe represent the coup injury. However, there may also be contusions of the frontal poles where the frontal lobe has struck the skull as a result of the forces inside the head; the frontal injuries are contrecoup contusions. Sometimes, contrecoup injury may occur in the absence of a visible coup injury.

Diffuse axonal injury. Acceleration/deceleration injury can stretch or tear nerve cell processes, causing a diffuse axonal injury. In severe damage, there is a permanent dementia.

Diffuse brain swelling. Such swelling is caused by oedema of the parenchyma together with congestion of cerebral blood vessels and it may follow injuries of many different kinds.

Neoplasms

The commonest neoplasms of the CNS are metastases from cancers elsewhere in the body. Common primary lesions include lung carcinoma, breast carcinoma, melanoma, leukaemia and lymphoma. Primary neoplasms of the CNS may be classified as benign or malignant, according to their histological appearances and degree of infiltration. Malignant tumours may produce secondary deposits within central nervous tissue but they metastasize outside the central nervous system only on exceptionally rare occasions. However, even benign neoplasms can cause death by compressing vital structures or causing herniation through their space-occupying effects.

57. Stroke

Questions
- What is the difference between ischaemic and haemorrhagic stroke?
- What are the risk factors for the development of stroke?
- What are the clinical sequelae of stroke?

The term stroke refers to the sudden onset of neurological symptoms caused by an intracerebral vascular event, which can be either infarction of part of the brain (ischaemic stroke) or haemorrhage (haemorrhagic stroke). Strokes are sometimes called cerebrovascular accidents.

Ischaemic stroke

Infarction from ischaemia accounts for approximately 80% of strokes. There are many causes, but these can be divided into three main groups: local arterial obstruction (the commonest), a generalized reduction in perfusion and local venous obstruction.

Local arterial obstruction causes infarction in the territory supplied by the obstructed artery if there is not an adequate collateral supply. For example, even if one internal carotid artery is occluded, the circle of Willis provides anastomotic connections that can allow adequate blood flow. This event is most likely if occlusion develops slowly, allowing the collateral vessels time to enlarge and compensate for the changed pattern of circulation. By comparison, the arteries within the brain parenchyma have poorly developed collaterals and are end-arteries. Causes of obstruction include:

- emboli, usually from atheromatous plaques of the proximal aorta or carotid arteries (Fig. 3.57.1) or from mural thrombi of left atrium or left ventricle; other sources include vegetations of the mitral or aortic valve, and fat embolism following major trauma
- atheroma of cerebral arteries, especially if complicated by thrombosis (Fig. 3.57.1)
- vasculitis.

A **generalized reduction in cerebral perfusion** can occur if systolic blood pressure falls or intercerebral pressure rises. Autoregulation normally keeps the cerebral blood flow relatively constant over a wide range of systemic arterial pressures. However, this flow will fall below a critical threshold and the blood supply will be inadequate if the systolic blood pressure falls below approximately 50 mmHg or if the intracerebral pressure rises to a level at which the arterial pressure cannot push blood into the cranial cavity. The neurons are most sensitive to hypoxia and are the first to suffer ischaemic injury. The **watershed areas** of the brain are particularly prone to hypoxia when there is global is-

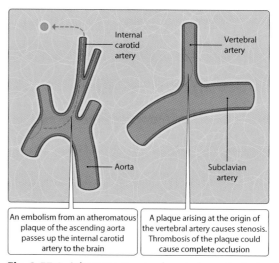

An embolism from an atheromatous plaque of the ascending aorta passes up the internal carotid artery to the brain

A plaque arising at the origin of the vertebral artery causes stenosis. Thrombosis of the plaque could cause complete occlusion

Fig. 3.57.1 Atheroma can produce ischaemic strokes in two ways: by acting as a source of emboli (A) or by directly obstructing the flow of blood (B).

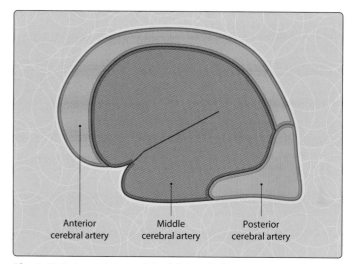

Anterior cerebral artery   Middle cerebral artery   Posterior cerebral artery

Fig. 3.57.2 Lateral view of the left hemisphere showing the territories supplied by the three major cerebral arteries. The borders between the territories are the watershed areas.

chaemia. The watershed zones represent the boundaries between arterial territories (Fig. 3.57.2). For example, the junction of the areas supplied by the anterior and middle cerebral arteries lies along the superior cerebral convexity. These zones are especially likely to become ischaemic if there is a failure of oxygenation either in hypotension (e.g. shock, arrhythmia) or in respiratory failure. The term 'watershed infarct' is used when these border areas become necrotic as a result.

Venous infarcts are blockage of the venous sinuses by thrombosis, which can occur as a complication of local sepsis or increased coagulability of the blood. Haemorrhagic necrosis of the brain follows.

Morphological changes

Morphological changes of infarction take time to develop. The neurons exhibit necrotic features in approximately 8 hours. After approximately 12 hours, neutrophils are seen infiltrating into the infarcted area. The tissue starts to soften and there is swelling and oedema of the infarct and surrounding tissue, which can have a space-occupying lesion effect. There may also be haemorrhage into the infarcted tissue; such haemorrhagic infarcts may come to resemble primary haemorrhagic strokes if there is extravasation of large amounts of blood. Approximately 3 days after the infarct, macrophages begin to infiltrate the lesion and phagocytose necrotic tissue. As this process proceeds, the tissue becomes soft and amorphous, producing the classic appearances of **liquefactive (colliquative) necrosis.** Healing is associated with absorption of liquefied tissue but a cyst-like cavity may remain (Fig. 3.57.3).

Clinical consequences

The symptoms and signs of ischaemic infarction are related to the site of tissue damage and whether brain herniation occurs owing to the space-occupying effect of the infarct.

The onset of cerebral infarction may be preceded by **transient ischaemic attacks (TIAs).** These events are defined as episodes of neurological dysfunction that completely resolve within 24 hours. They are caused by transient thrombi overlying plaques or by emboli that disappear sufficiently quickly that no irreversible neuronal injury occurs. Patients with TIAs are at high risk of developing a subsequent stroke.

Haemorrhagic stroke

Non-traumatic intracerebral haemorrhage is called haemorrhagic stroke. There are a number of causes.

Rupture of small vessel within brain. The most important predisposing factor is hypertension, which weakens the walls of small vessels, although the exact mechanism by which this produces brain haemorrhage is not fully understood. Other factors contributing to haemorrhagic stroke include anticoagulation therapy, coagulation disorders, vasculitis and amyloidosis. Haemorrhage can occur in many different sites, but the basal ganglia are most commonly affected.

Berry aneurysms. Saccular aneurysms of the arteries at the base of the brain are commonly called berry aneurysms. They develop at points of bifurcation (Fig. 3.57.4). Berry aneurysms result from a congenital weakness in the arterial wall. The aneurysm itself is not present at birth, however, because it takes some years for the aneurysm to develop and grow. Berry aneurysms are more common in individuals with polycystic kidney disease and coarctation of the aorta. Symptoms may be caused by pressure of the aneurysm on adjacent structures or by rupture, with haemorrhage into the subarachnoid space or into the brain parenchyma.

Vascular malformations. Most vascular malformations are congenital and include arteriovenous malformations and cavernous angiomas. These conditions are characterized by abnormal, dilated vessels, and they carry a risk of spontaneous haemorrhage, either into the brain parenchyma or the subarachnoid space.

Since haemorrhagic strokes cause disruption of brain tissue, brain swelling and herniation, the symptoms and signs are similar to those of ischaemic stroke. However, the onset of haemorrhagic stroke is often more sudden and dramatic, and it is more likely to be associated with severe headache.

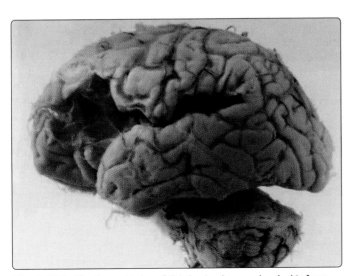

Fig. 3.57.3 The frontal lobe of this brain shows a healed infarct. The liquefactive necrosis has been absorbed, leaving a fluid-filled cavity lined by glial tissue.

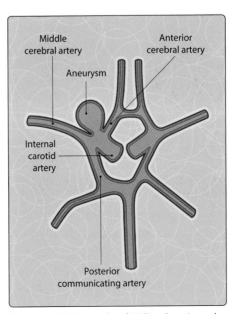

Fig. 3.57.4 The circle of Willis, showing a berry (saccular) aneurysm of the internal carotid artery arising at the junction with the anterior cerebral artery.

58. Alzheimer's disease

Questions
- What factors predispose to the development of Alzheimer's disease?
- What changes are seen in the brain in Alzheimer's disease?

Dementia can be defined as an acquired global impairment of cognitive function (i.e. the intellectual abilities involved in thinking, learning and remembering) with no decrease in the level of consciousness. There are many causes (Table 3.58.1), but by far the most common in industrialized countries is the topic of this chapter, Alzheimer's disease.

Morphological changes

The changes of Alzheimer's disease are found mainly in the cerebral cortex and limbic system. The feature most characteristic on macroscopic examination is atrophy of the cortex, most marked in the frontal and temporal lobes. The weight of the brain is reduced and there is compensatory dilatation of the ventricles. The amount of CSF increases to fill the extra space within the skull resulting from the decrease in the amount of brain tissue; this reactive increase in CSF is called secondary hydrocephalus, but note that CSF pressure remains normal.

Histologically, the hallmarks of Alzheimer's disease are:

- β-amyloid plaques
- neurofibrillary tangles
- loss of neurons
- deposition of β-amyloid around small vessels (amyloid angiopathy).

The plaques have a core of β-amyloid protein surrounded by dilated neuronal processes and reactive astrocytes. The neurofibrillary tangles are found within the cytoplasm of neurons and consist of corkscrew-like fibrils of tau, a microtubule-associated protein.

None of these changes is specific and they can all be found in elderly individuals without Alzheimer's disease. However, they are much more marked in patients with this condition.

Pathophysiology

Our understanding of the pathological mechanisms underlying Alzheimer's disease can be summarized in the amyloid β-protein cascade hypothesis (Fig. 3.58.1). According to this hypothesis, the initial defect is abnormal cleavage of a protein called amyloid precursor protein (APP), which is a normal transmembrane protein. This protein is normally degraded by proteolytic enzymes called secretases, but an insoluble fragment called the Aβ-peptide is produced if β-secretase followed by γ-secretase act on the APP molecule.

The Aβ-peptide tends to form β-pleated sheets, and thus accumulates as β- or Aβ-amyloid (Ch. 11). This amyloid forms the core of the plaques and is also deposited around small arterioles and capillaries, producing amyloid angiopathy. The plaques are associated with distortion and dilatation of neuronal processes, which could affect neural function (Fig. 3.58.2). The amyloid angiopathy causes ischaemia and haemorrhage, which could contribute to loss of neurons. Furthermore, β-amyloid may also have a direct toxic effect on neurons and be able to induce apoptosis; the generation of free radicals by β-amyloid has been implicated in some studies.

Tau protein forms neurofibrillary tangles when it becomes hyperphosphorylated (Fig. 3.58.2). The tangles of hyperphosphorylated tau have been shown to induce apoptosis and could, therefore, be a cause of neuronal loss. In addition, the hyperphosphorylated tau does not have normal biological activity and could adversely affect neuronal function. There is good evidence that Aβ-amyloid can be responsible for hyperphosphorylation of tau, but the mechanism is unclear and it is possible that other processes could also be at work. For example, there is an unusual frontotemporal dementia with parkinsonism linked to chromosome 17 (called FTDP-17) in which the dementia occurs with abnormalities in tau protein, caused by mutation of the gene for tau, but without β-amyloid deposits; this disease demonstrates that it is possible for tau protein abnormalities to cause dementia in the absence of β-amyloid.

Table 3.58.1 COMMON CAUSES OF DEMENTIA

Disorders	Examples
Primary neurodegenerative disorders	Alzheimer's disease; Pick's disease; Huntington's disease; diffuse Lewy body disease
Secondary dementias	
Cerebrovascular disease	Multi-infarct dementia
Prion diseases (spongiform encephalopathies)	Creutzfeld–Jacob disease; variant Creutzfeld–Jacob disease
Microorganisms	Neurosyphilis, HIV
Gross structural abnormalities	Hydrocephalus; space-occupying lesions
Metabolic abnormalities	Hypothyroidism; liver failure
Repeated diffuse trauma	Dementia pugilistica
Toxins	Chronic alcoholism; lead poisoning
Demyelinating diseases	Multiple sclerosis
Vitamin deficiencies	B_1, B_2, B_{12}

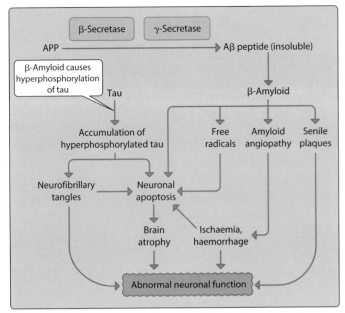

Fig. 3.58.1 Pathogenetic pathways in the development of Alzheimer's disease. APP, amyloid precursor protein.

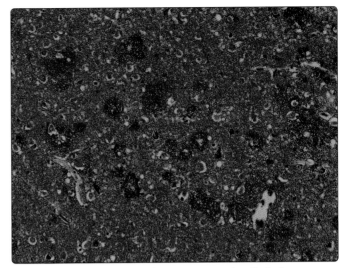

Fig. 3.58.2 A tissue section from a patient who died of Alzheimer's disease. Staining with a silver method shows senile plaques and neurofibrillary tangles. The former are more numerous in this section and are represented by the slightly poorly defined brown-black foci (these also contain Aβ-amyloid) while the latter are the much smaller and more well-defined black foci. Magnification ×200.

Genetic factors

A number of genes have been shown to be involved in Alzheimer's disease, and their contribution can be understood in terms of the amyloid β-protein cascade hypothesis.

Excessive production of amyloid precursor protein. The gene *APP* is found on chromosome 21 and so those with Down's syndrome (trisomy 21) have an extra copy of the gene *APP* and produce more APP and consequently more Aβ-amyloid. For this reason, most individuals with Down's syndrome over the age of 40 years develop Alzheimer's disease.

Mutated amyloid precursor protein. Mutations in *APP* can result in a form of early-onset familial Alzheimer's disease. The responsible mutations cause APP to be more prone to generate Aβ-amyloid.

Mutations affecting γ-secretase. Two related substances, presenilin-1 and presenilin-2, are components of γ-secretase; they are encoded by the genes *PSEN1* and *PSEN2*, respectively. Mutations of these genes are associated with increased Aβ-peptide production and cause a form of early-onset familial Alzheimer's disease.

Mutations affecting apolipoprotein E. The gene *APOE* codes for apolipoprotein E, which is involved in the redistribution of cholesterol during neuronal growth and injury and is found in the plaques of Alzheimer's disease. Individuals who have the allele ε4 (epsilon-4), which codes for the isoform E4, are more likely to develop Alzheimer's disease.

59. Osteoporosis and osteomalacia

Questions
- What is the difference between osteoporosis and osteomalacia?
- What are the causes of osteoporosis and osteomalacia?

Osteoporosis and osteomalacia are common conditions. Osteoporosis is a decrease in the mass of bone in the presence of normal mineralization, whereas osteomalacia is deficient mineralization of bone (Fig. 3.59.1).

Osteoporosis

Bone is constantly being remodelled by osteoblasts producing new bone and osteoclasts breaking it down. The pathogenesis of osteoporosis is an increase in bone resorption by osteoclasts over bone formation by osteoblasts.

Aetiology

There are many causes of osteoporosis, including disuse, loss of bone mass with age, increased circulating corticosteroids, hyperthyroidism, acromegaly, chronic renal failure, chronic liver failure, malnutrition and malabsorption. The first three of these account for the great majority of cases and are discussed below.

Disuse osteoporosis

Normal bone remodelling depends on the bone being subjected to the normal mechanical forces associated with movement and weight bearing. Therefore, if a body part is immobilized, the total mass of bone reduces. This condition is essentially a kind of disuse atrophy and produces localized osteoporosis. For example, there will be significant bone loss after a few weeks if a patient's arm is immobilized in plaster following a fracture. The mass of bone will return to normal after the fracture has healed, assuming normal activity of the limb is resumed.

A similar process affects astronauts subjected to long periods of weightlessness. In the microgravity of space, the weight that bones must support is reduced to almost zero and movement does not produce the same stresses as it would on Earth. The result is disuse osteoporosis; the high levels of serum calcium found in astronauts' blood during spaceflight reflects the increase in bone resorption over production.

Age-related osteoporosis

A systemic loss of bone mass with ageing is known as age-related osteoporosis, senile osteoporosis or, in females, postmenopausal osteoporosis.

The pathophysiology of age-related osteoporosis is not fully understood. However, an important factor determining whether it will become clinical problem in an individual is the **peak bone mass**. During early adulthood, the total mass of bone in the body reaches a peak (Fig. 3.59.2). After the age of approximately 30, it starts to decline as a predictable ageing phenomenon at a rate of approximately 0.7–1% per year. The total mass of bone in old age is thus a function of the peak bone mass that was achieved in early adulthood. Consequently, regular exercise before age 30 can protect against osteoporosis in later life by increasing peak bone mass.

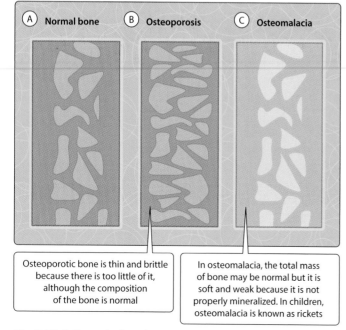

| Osteoporotic bone is thin and brittle because there is too little of it, although the composition of the bone is normal | In osteomalacia, the total mass of bone may be normal but it is soft and weak because it is not properly mineralized. In children, osteomalacia is known as rickets |

Fig. 3.59.1 Bone dysfunction.

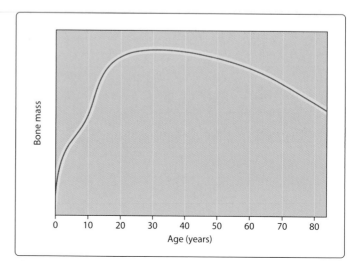

Fig. 3.59.2 Change in total bone mass with age in the human body.

After the menopause, the rate of bone loss in females accelerates because of the decrease in oestrogen production. The balance of cytokines in the bone is altered and there is an increase in osteoclastic activity. Consequently, women are more likely to suffer the effects of osteoporosis than men. Oestrogen replacement therapy protects against this cause of bone loss.

Another risk factor for osteoporosis is inadequate dietary calcium intake. The effect is especially important before age 30 years, probably because of the reduction in peak bone mass.

Corticosteroid-related osteoporosis

Glucocorticoids increase bone resorption and decrease bone formation. Therefore, osteoporosis is an important complication of long-term steroid therapy and is seen in Cushing's syndrome.

Clinical effects and diagnosis of osteoporosis

Osteoporotic bone is fragile and so it fractures with relatively minor trauma. The thinning of the bones may be visible on plain X-rays, but this feature is unreliable and only visible in advanced disease. Specialized imaging techniques (DEXA; dual energy X-ray absorptiometry) must be used to measure the amount of bone loss accurately.

Osteomalacia

Osteomalacia is decreased mineralization of bone matrix. The osteoid is laid down as normal but much of it remains unmineralized. The term **rickets** is used for the same condition in childhood; rickets is characterized by distinctive deformities of the growing skeleton.

Aetiology

Vitamin D deficiency

Vitamin D is obtained from the diet or from the conversion of precursors in the skin by ultraviolet light. The active metabolites of vitamin D (principally 1,25-dihydroxycholecalciferol, which is produced in the kidney) have important hormonal effects. In particular, 1,25-dihydroxycholecalciferol elevates plasma calcium and phosphate by increasing calcium and phosphate absorption from the intestine and increasing their retention by the kidney. It also promotes mineralization of newly formed osteoid. Lack of vitamin D owing to dietary deficiency, perhaps compounded by lack of exposure to sunlight, causes osteomalacia and rickets.

Malabsorption of calcium

Failure to absorb calcium from the small intestine is a common cause of osteomalacia and occasionally rickets. The underlying cause is usually coeliac disease, although other causes of malabsorption may also be responsible.

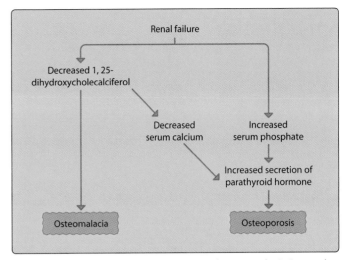

Fig. 3.59.3 Pathways to osteoporosis and osteomalacia in renal osteodystrophy.

Chronic renal failure

Most patients with long-standing renal failure have bone disease. The general term for bone disease in chronic renal failure is **renal osteodystrophy**; it is a complex condition that combines osteomalacia with hyperparathyroidism (Fig. 3.59.3). The renal failure is associated with reduction in 1,25-dihydroxycholecalciferol production, which causes a fall in serum calcium. The renal failure is also associated with phosphate retention and hyperphosphataemia, which further decreases the ionized fraction of plasma calcium. As a result of hypocalcaemia and hyperphosphataemia, there is secondary hyperparathyroidism. The net effect on the bones is that the lack of 1,25-dihydroxycholecalciferol causes osteomalacia, while the increase in parathyroid hormone tends to cause bone resorption and thus causes osteoporosis. There are also complex aberrations in bone remodelling that can even cause areas of increased bone density (**osteosclerosis**).

Inherited abnormalities of vitamin D metabolism

Inherited disorders of vitamin D metabolism are rare and present as rickets. Vitamin D supplementation has no effect, so these diseases are known as **vitamin D resistant rickets**.

Clinical features

Rickets produces bone deformities of varying types. A common feature is bowing of the long bones of the lower limbs because the abnormally soft bone is deformed by weight bearing.

In adults, osteomalacia commonly presents with bone pain and tenderness, which is most severe at sites of spontaneous incomplete stress fractures, visible radiologically as **Looser zones**, a characteristic feature of this disease. Muscle weakness is also common and appears to be related to vitamin D deficiency, although the pathophysiology is unclear. Skeletal deformities occur in severe osteomalacia.

60. Arthritis

Questions
- What are the most common forms of arthritis?
- What are the factors that predispose to the development of osteoarthritis?
- What are the extra-articular manifestations of rheumatoid disease?

Arthritis means inflammation of the joints. It is a common condition and there are many different aetiologies.

Osteoarthritis

Osteoarthritis is a very common condition that essentially results from degeneration of articular cartilage through wear and tear, although there are also genetic factors involved in its development. Eventually, the cartilage is worn away completely. The process is accelerated if there is previous joint damage or deformity of any type.

In the initial stages, the articular hyaline cartilage becomes soft and weak owing to an increased amount of water, decreased concentration of proteoglycans and weakening of collagen in the matrix. Chondrocytes adjacent to the bone proliferate and produce new matrix in an attempt to replace the abnormal cartilage, but eventually this process fails and the degenerative changes supervene.

Figure 3.60.1 shows some of the morphological changes in osteoarthritis. In the early stages, the surface of the hyaline cartilage becomes ragged and split, an appearance known as fibrillation. The subchondral bone becomes sclerotic through thickening of the bony trabeculae. Later, proliferation of bone at the edge of the joint produces irregular nodules called **osteophytes**. There is a chronic inflammatory infiltrate of the synovium and surrounding tissues, but it is not as marked as in rheumatoid arthritis. If the cartilage wears away completely, the underlying bone becomes polished smooth and comes to resemble ivory, a process known as eburnation. Cyst-like spaces form in the bone underlying the joint as synovial fluid is forced into it through microfractures.

Clinically, osteoarthritis typically affects the hips and knees, cervical vertebrae, hands and wrists. However, any joint can be affected, especially if it has been previously injured. Symptoms include pain, stiffness and swelling of the joint.

Gout

The deposition of urate crystals in the tissues causes gout. The main organs involved are the joints and kidneys. The most common clinical manifestation is arthritis; in 90% of those affected the great toe is involved.

Pathogenesis

Uric acid is a breakdown product of purine bases and is excreted via the kidneys. The levels circulating in the blood are rather variable, but increased amounts are associated with the risk of deposition of monosodium urate crystals in the tissues. Either overproduction of urate or reduced renal excretion can result in hyperuricaemia. In most cases, overproduction of urate is responsible, although the aetiology is unknown in the majority of patients. Occasionally, there is an identifiable cause, such as an inherited enzyme defect such as Lesch–Nyhan syndrome or increased cell turnover in diseases such as leukaemia causing increased formation of urate from the metabolism of purines in the malignant cells. The effects of urate depend on where it is deposited:

- **joint disease**: when deposited in the joints, monosodium urate crystals activate neutrophils causing intense acute inflammation; recurrent attacks produce joint deformity
- **skin and soft tissues**: if large amounts of urate accumulate, chalky deposits called gouty tophi form
- **kidney disease**: urate is readily precipitated in the relatively acid environment of the renal medulla and urinary passages, blocking tubules or forming stones; damage to the renal parenchyma may be sufficient to cause renal failure (gouty nephropathy), but this is usually only seen in severe cases (e.g. gout associated with leukaemia).

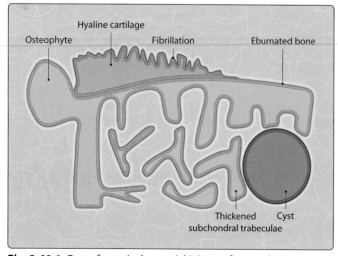

Fig. 3.60.1 Part of a typical synovial joint surface to show changes in osteoarthritis.

Rheumatoid arthritis

Rheumatoid arthritis is a systemic autoimmune disorder characterized by chronic synovitis. The arthritis is often severe and associated with a dense chronic inflammatory infiltrate of the synovium. A typical feature is **pannus**, a layer of inflamed granulation tissue growing over and destroying hyaline cartilage. There is also inflammation and fibrosis of adjacent bone, tendons and soft tissue. The overall effect is to produce severe pain and deformity. Eventually, the articular cartilage is destroyed and the pannus bridges the ends of the exposed bones. As the pannus matures into fibrous tissue, the ends of the bones become joined (fibrous ankylosis). Ultimately, the fibrous tissue ossifies and the joint becomes obliterated by bone (bony ankylosis).

There are a number of possible extra-articular manifestations of rheumatoid arthritis, for example vasculitis, chronic inflammatory nodules (rheumatoid nodules) in the skin and elsewhere, and serosal inflammation. In some cases the condition can overlap with other autoimmune disorders such as systemic lupus erythematosus.

There are a number of complex immunological abnormalities in patients with rheumatoid arthritis. One that is used in clinical diagnosis is the presence of **rheumatoid factor**, which is the name given to autoantibodies directed against the Fc portion of IgG. It is present in approximately 80% of those with rheumatoid arthritis, but it can also be found in other autoimmune diseases.

Clinically, rheumatoid arthritis is more common in females and its peak incidence is in young adults, although it can occur at any age. The arthritis tends to be symmetrical and commonly involves the hands and feet.

Seronegative arthritis

The seronegative arthritides are autoimmune diseases not associated with rheumatoid factor. They have a number of overlapping features, including an association with HLA-B27, the presence of an arthritis that has a tendency to involve the axial skeleton, and inflammation of tendinous attachments. Histologically, chronic inflammation of synovium and adjacent tissues is observed. The seronegative arthritides include ankylosing spondylitis, psoriatic arthritis (which occurs in approximately 10% of patients with psoriasis), autoimmune-mediated arthritis following an infection and arthritis associated with inflammatory bowel disease.

Infectious arthritis

There are many different organisms that can infect joints. They can be introduced into the joint in a number of ways (Fig. 3.60.2). Gonococci, staphylococci, streptococci, Gram-negative bacteria and *Haemophilus influenzae* produce a suppurative arthritis characterized clinically by the sudden onset of a hot, red, painful swollen joint with a restricted range of movement. The appearances seen under the microscope are typical of inflammation induced by pyogenic bacteria. Other infective arthritides include **Lyme disease**, which is caused by *Borrelia burgdorferi*, and **tuberculous arthritis**, caused by *Mycobacterium tuberculosis*.

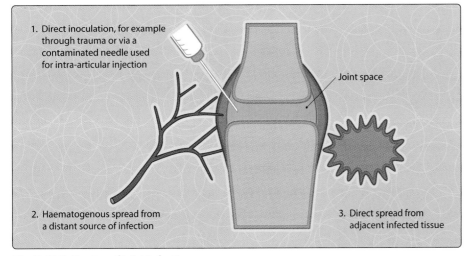

1. Direct inoculation, for example through trauma or via a contaminated needle used for intra-articular injection

Joint space

2. Haematogenous spread from a distant source of infection

3. Direct spread from adjacent infected tissue

Fig. 3.60.2 Routes of joint infection.

61. Endocrine pathology

Questions
- Which diseases can result from hyperplasia or atrophy of endocrine glands?
- What are the most common tumours that arise within the thyroid gland?
- What is Cushing's syndrome?

Much of the pathology of endocrine organs is related to hormone excess or deficiency. Typically, excess hormone production is associated with hyperplasia or neoplasia of the endocrine cells producing the hormone. Deficiency of a hormone is usually associated with atrophy of the endocrine cells or their destruction, depending on the pathogenesis.

Neoplasms of endocrine cells are common. They can secrete excess hormones, in which case they can manifest clinically through the hormone effects (Fig. 3.61.1A). Neoplasms that cause clinical effects by secreting excess hormones are called functioning tumours, while those that do not produce clinically apparent hormones are called non-functioning tumours. If a non-functioning tumour destroys the gland in which it has arisen, there may be a lack of hormone production and clinical presentation is with hormone deficiency (Fig. 3.61.1B). Endocrine neoplasms can also have non-endocrine effects (Fig. 3.61.1C).

Hyperplasia and atrophy of glandular tissue
Glands can be hyperplastic either because they are autonomously hyperactive or because they are being excessively stimulated by a stimulating factor. An example of the former is primary hyperparathyroidism. In this condition, primary hyperplasia of the parathyroid glands is associated with an autonomous increase in parathyroid hormone secretion. An example of excess stimulation by a factor produced outside the gland is Graves' disease, in which the thyroid-stimulating hormone (TSH) receptors on thyroid epithelial cells are abnormally stimulated by an autoantibody, causing enlargement of the thyroid gland and excess hormone production; the excess of thyroid hormone produces a constellation of clinical features called hyperthyroidism.

Although hyperplasia of glands is often associated with excess hormone production, it can occur without an excess of hormone production in some circumstances. For example, in iodine deficiency, the thyroid gland enlarges even though there is a deficiency in thyroid hormones (hypothyroidism). Iodine is required for the synthesis of thyroid hormones, so there is a failure of production of thyroid hormones in iodine-deficient individuals. One result of the reduced circulating levels of thyroid hormones is increased TSH production, because of decreased negative feedback on the pituitary gland. The increased TSH causes thyroid hyperplasia.

Atrophy of glandular tissue is usually a result of lack of a stimulating factor. For example, hypothyroidism caused by lack of TSH is associated with atrophy of the thyroid epithelium.

Damage to endocrine tissue
There are many different ways in which damage to endocrine cells can occur and hormone deficiency will result if the damage is sufficiently extensive. Important examples include autoimmune reactions, neoplasms (primary or secondary), infection,

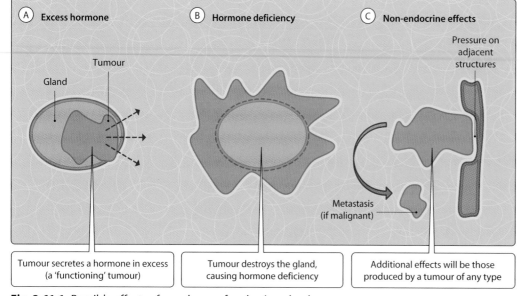

| A Excess hormone | B Hormone deficiency | C Non-endocrine effects |

Pressure on adjacent structures

Gland

Tumour

Metastasis (if malignant)

| Tumour secretes a hormone in excess (a 'functioning' tumour) | Tumour destroys the gland, causing hormone deficiency | Additional effects will be those produced by a tumour of any type |

Fig. 3.61.1 Possible effects of neoplasms of endocrine glands.

infarction, and surgical removal. To take the specific example of the adrenal gland, chronic adrenal insufficiency (Addison's disease) can be caused by autoimmune adrenalitis, metastases from carcinomas of the breast or lung, tuberculosis, infarction in severe septic shock, and bilateral adrenalectomy.

Endocrine neoplasms

There are a wide variety of endocrine neoplasms. Occasionally, they can occur as part of **multiple endocrine neoplasia** (MEN) syndromes, which are unusual conditions inherited as autosomal dominant traits and characterized by proliferative lesions affecting multiple endocrine organs.

Neuroendocrine neoplasms. This term is used for tumours that have membrane-bound neurosecretory granules, which can be demonstrated under the electron microscope. This group of tumours includes the carcinoids, which arise in the gastrointestinal tract (especially the appendix), lung and elsewhere. Carcinoids secrete serotonin (5-hydroxytryptamine), which occasionally causes flushing, diarrhoea, abdominal pain, breathlessness and fibrous thickening of the tricuspid and pulmonary valves (**carcinoid syndrome**). Other neuroendocrine tumours include islet cell tumours of the pancreas and medullary carcinoma of the calcitonin-secreting C-cells of the thyroid. The most aggressive type of neuroendocrine neoplasm is the **small cell carcinoma**. This lesion arises in the lung, gastrointestinal tract and elsewhere. It is considered to represent the most malignant end of the spectrum of neuroendocrine neoplasia.

Thyroid neoplasms. These are common lesions and include **adenomas** (benign) and **carcinomas** (malignant). There are four main types of carcinoma:
  – papillary carcinoma, the most common type, tends to remain localized to the thyroid and cervical nodes
  – follicular carcinoma, which often spreads through the blood and can present with skeletal metastases
  – medullary carcinoma, a neuroendocrine neoplasm
  – anaplastic carcinoma, rare and poor prognosis.

Pituitary neoplasms. Most pituitary tumours are adenomas. They may be functioning or non-functioning. Their growth within the pituitary fossa can have a number of mass effects (e.g. expansion and erosion of the sella turcica, visual field defects owing to pressure on the optic chiasm, and raised intracranial pressure). Functional lesions may present with hormonal effects, but if a non-functioning tumour destroys the normal pituitary cells the patient may present with hypopituitarism.

Adrenal neoplasms. Tumours of the adrenal cortex may be non-functioning or functioning. If the latter, they can secrete adrenocortical steroids such as cortisol, which produces Cushing's syndrome (see below). Tumours of catecholamine-secreting cells of the adrenal medulla are called **phaeochromocytomas**; the excess catecholamines produce hypertension.

Cushing's syndrome: an example of endocrine pathology

Cushing's syndrome is caused by excess corticosteroids. The clinical features include hypertension, weight gain, hyperglycaemia, osteoporosis, and depression, amongst others. It has a number of possible causes (Fig. 3.61.2):

■ **excess adrenocorticotrophic hormone (ACTH) production** by an adenoma of the pituitary or by some other neoplasm (e.g. lung carcinoma); the excess hormone production is associated with hyperplasia of the adrenal glands on account of the excessive stimulation by ACTH

■ **autonomous excess secretion** of hormone by the gland itself caused by a functioning neoplasm of the adrenal gland or primary adrenocortical nodular hyperplasia (pathogenesis obscure); negative feedback by the excess cortisol on the pituitary will result in low ACTH concentrations

■ **steroid therapy**: if a patient takes high doses of steroids, features of Cushing's syndrome result; negative feedback causes ACTH concentrations to fall and the adrenal cortex becomes atrophic.

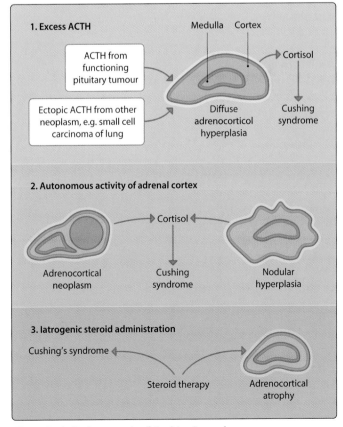

Fig. 3.61.2 Pathogenesis of Cushing's syndrome.

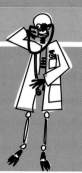

Glossary

Abbreviations

CT	computed tomography
H&E	haematoxylin and eosin stain
HIV	human immunodeficiency virus
HLA	human leukocyte antigen
IL	interleukin
MRI	magnetic resonance imaging
NSAID	non-steroidal anti-inflammatory drug
Th1 and Th2	T helper type 1 or 2 (cells)
TNF	tumour necrosis factor

Terms

Abscess
A localized collection of pus

Aetiology
A cause, e.g. of a disease process

Anaemia
Reduced blood haemoglobin concentration

Anastomosis
A connection between two hollow structures (e.g. two blood vessels), which may be physiological or pathological in nature

Arrhythmia
An abnormal heart rhythm, which may lead to significant reduction in or complete loss of cardiac output

Asymptomatic
The state of having no symptoms

Auscultation
Listening to a part of the body (most commonly the chest or abdomen) using a stethoscope

Cachexia
Extreme weight loss

Chemotherapy
Usually used to describe forms of systemic drug treatment for cancer and deliverable by a variety of routes but most commonly given as tablets or an intravenous infusion. Chemotherapy is usually given for white blood cell-derived cancers (e.g. leukaemia) or to treat a solid organ cancer that has developed widespread growth to distant sites within the body

Constitutional symptoms
Non-specific symptoms such as nausea, poor appetite, fever and weight loss

Cytopathology
A clinical pathology specialty involving examination of a sample comprising individual cells or small clusters of cells that have been removed from the body by scraping (e.g. cervical smear) or fine needle aspiration (see below; e.g. pleural fluid, a thyroid or breast mass). Diagnosis is based mainly on the characteristics of these individual cells or cell clusters

Digital rectal examination
Examination of the lower rectum and prostate gland by introducing a gloved index finger into the rectum via the anal canal

Dysfunction
Loss of normal function

Epidemiology
A study of the patterns of disease incidence and prevalence across on a global basis

Extracellular
Outside a cell or cells

Fine needle aspiration (FNA)
A means of obtaining a sample of cells for cytological examination by applying suction (usually with a syringe) to a small-diameter needle that is inserted into an organ, tissue or a body cavity containing fluid

Fistula
An abnormal connection (usually lined by granulation tissue) between two epithelial-lined surfaces

Gram stain
A staining method used on tissue sections or microbiological samples and enabling a basic division of bacteria into Gram-positive and Gram-negative types; this is an important component of the classification system for bacteria

Granulation tissue
Loose connective tissue containing inflammatory cells and delicate capillaries and representing a stage in the reaction to a tissue injury

Granuloma
A localized collection of macrophages

Haematoxylin and eosin (H&E) stain
The most common 'routine' staining method used in diagnostic histopathology practice for tissue sections. Haematoxylin is a blue stain that highlights nucleic acids and, therefore, stains nuclei. Eosin is an orange-pink stain that highlights cellular cytoplasm and extracellular tissue components such as collagen

Haematuria
Blood within the urine; it may be visible only under microscopic examination or to the naked eye

Haemolysis
Breakdown of red blood cells with release of haemoglobin

Heterotopic
The presence of a tissue at an abnormal site, e.g. heterotopic bone within an old scar

Histopathology
A clinical pathology specialty involving examination of cells within the overall structure of the tissue section being examined, e.g. sections obtained at an endoscopic procedure or a surgical operation

Homeostasis
The maintenance of a steady and balanced state: when all of the anatomical, biological and physiological mechanisms within the body are working normally

Hyper-
A prefix describing a state in which a variable is higher than the normal value (e.g. hypertension, high blood pressure)

Hypo-
A prefix describing a state in which a variable is lower than the normal value (e.g. hypotension, low blood pressure)

Immunosuppression
A term that is essentially synonymous with 'immunodeficiency' and which describes a state in which the function of the immune system is reduced, either by a primary disease or by a treatment

Infarction
Necrosis following ischaemia

Intracellular
Within a cell or cells

Ischaemia
A state characterized by a low oxygen tension, e.g. within a tissue

Isotope body scan
A means of looking for distant metastases of a cancer; it involves the injection of a radioactive isotope into the body and then imaging with a special detection system to identify the radioactivity concentrated in tumour deposits

Leukocyte
A white blood cell; 'leukocytosis' refers to the presence of increased numbers of circulating white blood cells within the blood or a solid tissue

Lumen
The space within a hollow organ, e.g. within the intestine

Macroscopic appearance
Appearance to the naked eye

-megaly
Enlargement of an organ, e.g. splenomegaly

Melaena
Black sticky stools containing haemoglobin breakdown products and usually caused by a haemorrhage into the upper gastrointestinal tract

Needle core biopsy
A means of obtaining a tissue sample for histopathological examination by introducing a needle (with a greater diameter than that used in fine needle aspiration) into an organ or tissue that can 'cut' a cylinder of tissue out of the structure

Pathological
A process occurring abnormally within the body, i.e. as part of a disease

Perfusion
Blood supply to an organ or tissue

Perl's stain
A tissue section staining method relying on the Prussian blue chemical reaction and used to demonstrate the presence of iron

Presymptomatic
The state in which an individual has an (early) disease process that has not (yet) produced symptoms

Physiological
A process occurring as a normal event within the body

Radiotherapy
Forms of treatment for cancer based on delivery of ionizing radiation to a tissue or organ; it is usually a localized rather than systemic treatment and may represent the main treatment modality or part of a complex treatment (e.g. with surgery and/or chemotherapy)

Sinus
A tract lined with granulation tissue connecting an abscess cavity with an epithelial-lined surface

Stem cell
A primitive cell type that has the capacity to undergo cell division and to develop (differentiate) into one or more mature cell types; stem cells are essential to enable the repopulation of tissues as a component of normal cell and tissue turnover

Stenosis
Narrowing, e.g. of a blood vessel or a component of the gastrointestinal tract

Tachycardia
An increased pulse rate

T helper cells
Subsets of T lymphocytes; Th1 cells help to orchestrate cellular immunity while Th2 cells promote humoral immunity

Ulcer
A defect in an epithelial surface or lining

Ultrasound
Very-high-frequency sound waves used in body imaging

Viscus
An internal organ

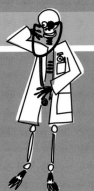

Index